Biological Aspects of Suicidal Behavior

Advances in Biological Psychiatry

Vol. 30

Series Editors

W.P. Kaschka Ulm/Ravensburg
W.F. Gattaz São Paulo

Biological Aspects of Suicidal Behavior

Volume Editors

W.P. Kaschka Ulm/Ravensburg

D. Rujescu Halle

4 figures, 4 in color, and 6 tables, 2016

KARGER Basel · Freiburg · Paris · London · New York · Chennai · New Delhi · Bangkok · Beijing · Shanghai · Tokyo · Kuala Lumpur · Singapore · Sydney

Advances in Biological Psychiatry

Prof. Dr. Wolfgang P. Kaschka
Department of Psychiatry I
University of Ulm
ZfP Südwürttemberg
Weingartshofer Strasse 2
DE–88190 Ravensburg (Germany)

Prof. Dr. Dan Rujescu
Klinik und Poliklinik für Psychiatrie,
Psychotherapie und Psychosomatik
der Martin-Luther Universität
Halle-Wittenberg
Julius-Kühn-Strasse 7
DE–06112 Halle/Saale (Germany)

Library of Congress Cataloging-in-Publication Data

Biological aspects of suicidal behavior / volume editors, W.P. Kaschka, D. Rujescu.
p. ; cm. -- (Advances in biological psychiatry, ISSN 0378-7354 ; vol. 30)
Includes bibliographical references and index.
ISBN 978-3-318-05583-2 (hard cover : alk. paper) -- ISBN 978-3-318-05584-9 (electronic version)
I. Kaschka, Wolfgang P., editor. II. Rujescu, D. (Dan), editor. III. Series: Advances in biological psychiatry ; v. 30. 0378-7354
[DNLM: 1. Depression--drug therapy. 2. Suicide--psychology. 3. Adrenergic Neurons--physiology. 4. Mental Disorders--genetics. W1 AD44 v.30 2016 / WM 165]
RC569
362.28--dc23

2015032176

Bibliographic Indices. This publication is listed in bibliographic services, including Current Contents® and Index Medicus.

www.karger.com
Printed in Germany on acid-free and non-aging paper (ISO9706) by Kraft Druck, Ettlingen
ISSN 0378–7354
e-ISSN 1662–2774
ISBN 978–3–318–05583–2
e-ISBN 978–3–318–05584–9

Contents

Immunology

Treatment

Outlook

Preface

According to a definition of the Institute of Medicine of the National Academies of the USA [1], suicide is 'a fatal self-inflicted destructive act with explicit or inferred intent to die'. Globally, year by year, approximately one million people die by suicide, which corresponds to a rate of 16 per 100,000. In the year 2012, suicide accounted for 1.4% of all deaths worldwide, making it the fifteenth leading cause of death throughout the lifespan and the second leading cause of death among 15- to 29-year-olds [2]. In Germany, the suicide rate as of 2013 is almost twice as high as the death rate from traffic accidents [3]. Therefore, effective and evidence-based interventions should be implemented at population, subpopulation, and individual levels to prevent suicides and suicide attempts. However, the reliable assessment of suicide risk in an individual person is a major scientific challenge. Although apparently relevant, psychological, psychosocial, and cultural factors offer merely weak predictive power with regard to suicidal behaviour, and even the clinical history of a patient, though extremely valuable, can be non-specific. It is generally accepted that mental disorders per se represent a risk factor for suicidal behaviour, but there appear to exist other causative factors – environmental as well as dispositional – which are independent of psychiatric diseases. During recent years, an increasing amount of research has been dedicated to the analysis of the neurobiological basis of suicide, enabling the development of neuro-psycho-biological models which may help to improve our understanding of this complex behaviour. This book provides a comprehensive overview on the epidemiological, neurobiological, and psychopharmacological aspects of suicide and suicide attempts throughout the lifespan.

Värnik and Wasserman present a meticulous review of the worldwide epidemiology of completed and attempted suicide. Mainly based on data from the World Health Organization, they draw our attention to the broad spectrum of factors influencing suicide rates, among which age and gender are only the most prominent ones. In addition, among others, societal, cultural, socioeconomic, and geographic effects have been identified. Methodological problems involved in the recording of suicide and attempted suicide rates are also discussed.

The important issue of suicidal ideation, suicide attempts, and completed suicide in adolescents is dealt with in the chapter by Sarchiapone, D'Aulerio and Iosue, with special emphasis on neurobiological aspects. The authors review alterations in major neurotransmitter and signalling systems found to be related to suicidal behaviour. Most interestingly, different results have been obtained in a number of parameters when groups of adolescents and adults were compared. In many cases, the biological significance of these differences has yet to be revealed.

A great number of clinical as well as post-mortem brain studies have shown neurobiological abnormalities associated with suicidal behaviour. Many of these were pointed out to be related to the serotonergic and noradrenergic neurotransmitter systems. The role of these systems, their intracellular signalling pathways and downstream effector molecules and their effects on the regulation of target genes in suicidal behaviour are discussed in the chapter by Dwivedi.

Among neurotransmitter systems, special attention has focused on the role of GABA in depression and suicide. Pabba and Sibille review the current evidence – mainly from post-mortem studies – suggesting a dysfunction of GABAergic systems in suicide victims having suffered from major depressive disorder (MDD-related suicides) compared to those not having suffered from major depression (MDD-unrelated suicides).

Giegling and Rujescu focus on the genetic part of suicidal behaviour. Beside medical, psychological, psychosocial, social, cultural, and socioeconomic parameters, biological factors, especially genetic variants, were also shown to be risk factors for suicidal behaviour. The heritability is about 55% assuming a polygenic risk model. The chapter gives an overview on first-candidate gene studies focusing mainly on the serotonergic system. Additionally, newly started genome-wide association studies are discussed.

The relative contributions of heritable versus environmental risk factors to suicidal behaviour have become a more and more challenging question. In their chapter, Mandelli and Serretti provide a comprehensive overview on studies regarding the interaction between genes modulating brain functions and stressful life events in the aetiology of suicide.

A great number of studies have confirmed an association between early-life adversity and increased suicide risk. Turecki describes how epigenetic mechanisms induced by early-life adversity are able to mediate altered behavioural development, resulting in increased vulnerability toward psychopathology in general and suicidal behaviour in particular.

In an analysis of what might predispose individuals to make a suicide attempt or completed suicide, neurocognitive processes appear to play a crucial role. Richard-Devantoy and Courtet review evidence from the current literature showing that, in addition to impulsive aggression and persistent hopelessness, impairments in cognitive domains may increase the vulnerability to suicidal behaviour.

Clinical electrophysiology, although mostly neglected in earlier reviews, has also contributed to our knowledge on the neurobiological basis of suicide. For example, it was shown that the habituation of P300, an event-related potential, differed between patients with MDD *and* a history of suicidal behaviour and MDD patients *without* such a history. Hodgkinson, Steyer, Kaschka, and Jandl summarize recent electrophysiological studies and discuss their implications for suicide risk assessment and suicide prophylaxis.

The rapid development of neuroimaging techniques during the last decades has provided us with tools that allow the investigation of suicidal behaviour in vivo. Results obtained using the different methods of structural and functional neuroimaging are reviewed by Jollant. Derived from the data presented in the context of the current literature, the author proposes a neurocognitive model of suicidal behaviour which could stimulate the development of interventions for the prevention of suicide.

In recent years, evidence has accumulated indicating that inflammatory processes and alterations within the immune system may contribute to the pathophysiology not only of depression but also of suicidal behaviour. Postolache, Manalai, Brenner, and Brundin give a comprehensive overview of the available data and delineate novel strategies of intervention, targeting immune dysregulation and aiming at the improvement of suicide risk assessment and suicide prevention.

The topic of pharmacological influences on suicidal ideation and behaviour is addressed by Müller-Oerlinghausen and Lewitzka. Whereas a large variety of pharmacologically different compounds is able to induce depressive states, suicidal ideation and suicidal behaviour, pharmaceutical agents that effectively counteract suicidality are surprisingly rare. Over the years, satisfactory evidence of an antisuicidal efficacy has been presented for lithium salts and clozapine only. The authors provide a comprehensive review of the literature, also covering the question of possible mechanisms of action. As for lithium, in addition to studies based on the use of lithium salts as pharmaceutical drugs, some studies have been published on the potential antisuicidal effects of lithium as a trace element in drinking water. These are also critically discussed.

Rujescu, Kaschka and Kaschka outline possible further directions of research which might be promising to improve our understanding of the neurobiological foundations of suicidal behaviour. It is suggested that biological parameters should be integrated into algorithms for the assessment of suicide risk in individual persons. Thereby, neurobiological research can be expected to make a significant contribution to personalized medicine in general and to suicide prevention in particular.

Wolfgang P. Kaschka, Ulm/Ravensburg
Dan Rujescu, Halle

References

1 The Institute of Medicine of the National Academies of the USA. http://www.nap.edu/author/IOM/institute-of-medicine (accessed March 10, 2015).

2 World Health Organization: Suicide Prevention (SUPRE). http://www.who.int/mental_health/prevention/suicide/suicideprevent/en/ (accessed March 10, 2015).

3 Statistisches Bundesamt: Todesursachenstatistik. http://www.gbe-bund.de (Suizid-Tabellen-Sterbefälle; accessed March 10, 2015).

Kaschka WP, Rujescu D (eds): Biological Aspects of Suicidal Behavior.
Adv Biol Psychiatry. Basel, Karger, 2016, vol 30, pp 1–10 (DOI: 10.1159/000435765)

Global Suicide

Peeter Värnik[a] • Danuta Wasserman[b–e]

[a]Estonian-Swedish Mental Health and Suicidology Institute (ERSI), Tallinn, Estonia; [b]Department of Psychiatry and Suicidology, [c]National Centre for Prevention of Suicide and Mental Ill-Health (NASP) and [d]Methods Development and Training in Suicide Prevention, WHO Collaborating Centre for Research, Karolinska Institute, Stockholm, Sweden; [e]European Psychiatric Association, Strasbourg, France

Abstract

Suicide is a serious public health problem worldwide. The suicide rate, i.e. the number of suicides per 100,000 of population, is considered to be an important indicator of national mental health and general well-being of society. The prevalence of suicide is often underestimated due to cultural, political and economic circumstances. The number of suicides in the world was estimated to be 804,000 in 2012, according to the WHO global suicide report. The age-standardized global suicide mortality rate was 11.4 per 100,000, accounting for 1.4% of all deaths. The highest crude suicide rate was in South Korea (36.6). In developed countries, male suicides have traditionally outnumbered female suicides. In 2012, the highest male-to-female suicide rate ratios (over 5.0) were found in Eastern Europe and the lowest in China (under 1.0). The risk to die by suicide increases with age. Notably, however, females in the age group 15–29 years had the highest suicide rate of all age groups in India and Latin America. The WHO estimates that for each adult suicide there may have been more than 20 others attempting suicide. Suicide risk is much higher in individuals who previously made a suicide attempt and research shows that suicide attempt is the single most important predictor of death by suicide. In suicide prevention work, strategies can be directed to the health care services or at the general population. A great need for preventive strategies for young people has been identified by the WHO. Therefore, an evidence school-based preventive method called Youth Aware of Mental Health (YAM) directed towards the entire classroom was developed in the EU-funded project 'Saving and Empowering Young Lives in Europe'.

Suicide is a serious public health problem worldwide. The negative effects are magnified manifold due to several reasons. Suicide not only concerns the deceased person but also affects family members, friends and colleagues several years after the event, sometimes throughout life. Every suicide death is premature and the average age at death is much lower in comparison with other causes of death. The proportion of potential years of life lost due to suicide is several times higher than the proportion of suicide deaths. Suicides are massively outnumbered by suicide attempts, which may cause serious injury and long-term disability. Therefore, in addition to human suffering, large economic costs are involved.

Although the decision to kill oneself is made on a very personal level, for more than a century it has been acknowledged as a social act [1] that can be investigated at societal levels. Suicide is often considered an important indicator of national mental health, reflecting the general well-being of the respective society.

Suicide is commonly measured in cases per 100,000 of inhabitants. Ideally, the rate is calculated as cases divided by person-years but the latter are seldom available, so mid-year counts of the population, or sometimes even the beginning-of-year population, are considered to be a close approximation. In addition to crude death rates, it is possible to calculate age-adjusted rates if mortality data are available by age groups. This eliminates the effects of population age structure, thereby facilitating an improved comparison between regions and over time. There are several versions of standardized populations used for calculating rates and the choice of method for standardization slightly affects the numerical outcome.

The prevalence of suicide is often underestimated due to cultural, political and economic circumstances. It may be reported under other subcategories of external causes of death, the most likely being death by injury of undetermined intent. Underestimations differ by method, e.g. suicide by hanging or firearm has better validity than suicide by poisoning or drowning because it is much harder to determine the intent for the latter.

Suicide Mortality Rates

Worldwide data about suicide mortality are improving year by year and this development is reflected in the WHO mortality databases. The latest achievement was the comprehensive WHO report 'Preventing Suicide: A Global Imperative' published in the second half of 2014 [2]. An impressive list of international contributors and working group members chaired by Phillips, Wasserman, Berman and De Leo created an overview of the current status of suicide and its prevention in the world. Annex A of the report, compiled by the Epidemiology Working Group (Phillips, Ajdacic-Gross, Carli, Corcoran, Crosby, De Leo, Gunnell, and Simon) includes best estimates of suicide data for 172 countries, including some demographic characteristics, and is therefore used as the source for the current chapter. The tables in this chapter include data from 104 countries with vital registration.

The number of suicides in the world was estimated to be 804,000 in 2012, according to the WHO report [2]. It is less than the frequently quoted 1 million cases per year and also much less than the 1.5 million cases that were predicted in 2002 by the WHO for 2020 [3]. It is extremely positive that this trend, which seemed to be going upward at the end of the 20th century, has reversed in many parts of the world. The age-standardized global suicide mortality rate was 11.4 per 100,000, accounting for 1.4% of all deaths. The largest number of suicides occurred in India, where estimates

Table 1. Top 20 countries according to the age-standardized suicide rate per 100,000 in 2012

Rank	Country	Quality level of data	Part of the world	Number of suicides	Crude suicide rate	Age-standardized suicide rate
1	Guyana	2	America S	277	34.8	44.2
2	South Korea	1	Asia W Pacific	17,908	36.6	28.9
3	Sri Lanka	2	Asia S	6,170	29.2	28.8
4	Lithuania	1	Europe E	1,007	33.3	28.2
5	Suriname	1	America S	145	27.2	27.8
6	Kazakhstan	1	Asia C	3,912	24.0	23.8
7	India	3	Asia S	258,075	20.9	21.1
8	Turkmenistan	2	Asia C	1,003	19.4	19.6
9	Russia	1	Europe E	31,997	22.4	19.5
10	Hungary	1	Europe E	2,519	25.3	19.1
11	Japan	1	Asia W Pacific	29,442	23.1	18.5
12	Belarus	1	Europe E	2,051	21.8	18.3
13	Ukraine	1	Europe E	9,165	20.1	16.8
14	Poland	2	Europe E	7,848	20.5	16.6
15	Latvia	1	Europe E	419	20.4	16.2
16	Montenegro	2	Europe E	117	18.9	15.3
17	Finland	1	Europe N	901	16.7	14.8
18	Belgium	1	Europe W	1,955	17.7	14.2
19	Iceland	1	Europe N	49	15.1	14.0
20	Moldova	1	Europe E	566	16.1	13.7

S = South; W = west; E = east; C = central; N = north.

show 258,000 persons died by suicide in 2012, accounting for 32% of all world suicides. The highest crude suicide rate in 2012 – 36.6 per 100,000 – was in South Korea. This number reflects the proportion of the population lost by suicide regardless of age. The age-standardized suicide rate, which is the best-suited indicator to make international comparisons, was highest in Guyana – 44.2 per 100,000 (table 1).

The WHO has measured suicide mortality rates since 1950 – shortly after its creation in 1948. The list of countries which have been leading in suicide rates in the world is not long. Japan had the highest suicide rate in the 1950s, while Hungary was the top country for the following three decades, followed by Lithuania from the early 1990s for another two decades [4]. Recently, Korea became the leading country with the highest suicide rate in the world.

Although available data on suicide are scarce for the years preceding the 1950s, a decrease from high levels of suicide morality during the 1930s and 1940s was observed in Switzerland, indicating they could have had the highest global suicide rate prior to that time period [5]. Contrary to the WHO figures, it has been estimated that the suicide rate in Sri Lanka reached 47 cases per 100,000 in the first half of the 1990s [6], which would make it the leading country with the highest suicide rate between the 'Hungarian period' and the 'Lithuanian period'.

Suicide has been in a preventive focus in Finland and Denmark but even when the rates surpassed 30 per 100,000 they were dwarfed by more extreme rates in Hungary during the same period. Similarly, very high suicide rates in Russia, Latvia and Estonia were overshadowed by those of Lithuania [4].

The earliest statistical reports on suicide rates date back to the mid-19th century. There is notable variability in developmental patterns of individual countries. During the past 150 years, the suicide rate in the USA has fluctuated between 10 and 15 per 100,000 and there does not seem to be a clear trend [7]. The suicide rate in Russia showed only a slight increase for one century from its first known level of 2.9 per 100,000 in 1838 but increased rapidly thereafter to one of the highest suicide mortality rates in the world [8]. Thomas and Gunnell [9] analysed suicide rates in England and Wales from 1861 to 2007. The suicide rate for males (30.3 per 100,000) peaked in 1905 and 1934 and has been declining since then. The female suicide rate peaked in the 1960s (11.8 per 100,000) and has also been declining since then.

An analysis of Swiss suicide data by Ajdacic-Gross et al. [5] covering the period 1881–2000 found that the male suicide rate peaked in the 1930s, while the rates for females peaked a decade later. Both line shapes yielded a low in the 1890s and in the 1960s. Condorelli [10] analysed Italian suicide rates from 1864 to 2005 and found that they rose from 2 per 100,000 in the beginning of the study period to over 10 in the 1930s and declined after that, never reaching the previous high. In Denmark, Paerregaard [11] found that the suicide rate was relatively high in 1861 (29.9 per 100,000) but declined to 12.8 in 1918, only to show an increasing trend in 1976 (26.0 per 100,000). In the 1980s, however, it started to decline again.

At a broader regional level, however, a clear pattern emerges. Evidence shows that during the last 60 years the heart of the problem of suicide mortality has shifted from Western Europe to Eastern Europe and now to Asia [4]. It may take another decade but there are some signs that it may next move on to Latin America.

The Proportion of Male and Female Suicides

Male suicides have outnumbered female suicides in nearly all regions and countries for which data are available. In 2012, among the 172 member states of the WHO with populations over 300,000, the mean male-to-female gender ratio (M/F ratio) was 3.2 according to the WHO report [2]. The M/F ratio in the world was also 3.2 in the 1950s but by the turn of the 21st century it had increased to 3.6 and further growth was predicted [3]. This did not happen and with hindsight it appears that the temporary increase was primarily caused by political changes in Eastern Europe.

There are clear gender differences observed between world regions in relation to suicidality. In 2012, data show that the highest M/F ratios were found in Eastern European countries, commonly over 5.0 (table 2), and the lowest in Asian countries – under 2.0 (China notably under 1.0). In developed countries, the ratio was between

Table 2. Top 20 and bottom 10 countries according to the male-to-female age-standardized suicide rate ratio in 2012 in comparison with 2000

Rank of M/F ratio, 2012	Country	Part of the world	Year 2012			Year 2000			Ratio change, 2000 to 2012
			suicide rate, male	suicide rate, female	M/F rate ratio	suicide rate, male	suicide rate, female	M/F rate ratio	
1	Malta	Europe S	11.1	0.7	15.9	9.8	2.2	4.5	11.4
2	Belize	America C	4.9	0.5	9.8	7.3	0.6	12.2	–2.4
3	Morocco	Africa Arab	9.9	1.2	8.3	4.2	1.3	3.2	5.0
4	Poland	Europe E	30.5	3.8	8.0	33.8	4.8	7.0	1.0
5	Slovakia	Europe E	18.5	2.5	7.4	21.8	4.3	5.1	2.3
6	Latvia	Europe E	30.7	4.3	7.1	52.8	9.3	5.7	1.5
7	Barbados	America Carib.	4.1	0.6	6.8	6.0	1.0	6.0	0.8
8	Estonia	Europe E	24.9	3.8	6.6	43.6	9.5	4.6	2.0
9	Romania	Europe E	18.4	2.9	6.3	19.4	3.6	5.4	1.0
10	Panama	America C Latin	8.1	1.3	6.2	10.8	1.6	6.8	–0.5
11	Lithuania	Europe E	51.0	8.4	6.1	79.3	15.0	5.3	0.8
12	Ukraine	Europe E	30.3	5.3	5.7	54.5	9.1	6.0	–0.3
13	Georgia	Europe E	5.7	1.0	5.7	7.6	1.4	5.4	0.3
14	Russia	Europe E	35.1	6.2	5.7	64.3	9.6	6.7	–1.0
15	Armenia	Europe E	5.0	0.9	5.6	5.9	1.0	5.9	–0.3
16	Czech Rep.	Europe E	21.5	3.9	5.5	23.0	5.2	4.4	1.1
17	Cyprus	Europe S	7.7	1.5	5.1	1.5	1.1	1.4	3.8
18	Belarus	Europe E	32.7	6.4	5.1	66.2	8.8	7.5	–2.4
19	Costa Rica	America C Latin	11.2	2.2	5.1	12.1	1.8	6.7	–1.6
20	Moldova	Europe E	24.1	4.8	5.0	28.9	4.0	7.2	–2.2
95	Singapore	Asia SE	9.8	5.3	1.8	14.7	7.7	1.9	–0.1
96	Maldives	Asia S	7.8	4.9	1.6	23.3	18.3	1.3	0.3
97	India	Asia S	25.8	16.4	1.6	26.2	20.3	1.3	0.3
98	Brunei	Asia SE	7.7	5.2	1.5	6.8	4.2	1.6	–0.1
99	Haiti	America Carib.	3.3	2.4	1.4	3.8	2.5	1.5	–0.1
100	Albania	Europe S	6.6	5.2	1.3	8.5	5.6	1.5	–0.2
101	Kuwait	Asia Arab	1.0	0.8	1.3	1.4	1.3	1.1	0.2
102	Jordan	Asia Arab	2.2	1.9	1.2	2.7	2.1	1.3	–0.1
103	China	Asia W Pacific	7.1	8.7	0.8	17.4	21.7	0.8	0.0
104	Iraq	Asia Arab	1.2	2.1	0.6	1.0	1.9	0.5	0.0

Carib. = Caribbean (for other abbreviations, see table 1 footnote).

3.0 and 4.0. This general pattern has persisted for a longer period, even so long that Kushner [12] referred to several authors from the 19th century who state that the earliest statistics showed that approximately 3 out of every 4 completed suicides in both Europe and North America were found among males.

Many different causes have been offered to explain the persistent gender difference. Mościcki [13] named four based on suicidal behaviour in the USA, three of which have gained wider acceptance: lethality, alcohol abuse and socialization. Men tend to choose more lethal methods for suicide [14], perhaps more so in Europe than in the USA [15]. Large-scale intentional pesticide self-poisoning in economically less developed countries is partly the reason behind lower M/F ratios there [16]. A clear link between suicide and alcohol abuse has been found in several cultural settings, most notably in Western Europe [17], Eastern Europe and Russia [18]. The effect is stronger among males. Rapid social changes and perceived reduction in social role opportunities for men lead to social exclusion [19].

Age Patterns

The risk to die by suicide increases with age. However, variability in suicide rates by age in different countries is great. Trying to apply a systematic approach, Girard [20] described four different age patterns and showed how each of these is typical of a certain level of societal development. In most developed countries, the age curve peaks in the elderly, while in the countries with lower development levels the age curve peaks in adolescents and young adults. In countries with an intermediate level of development, the age curve is bimodal, with peaks among middle-aged adults and the elderly. In some of the most developed countries, which are able to provide a comfortable retirement, the age curve is convex, with a decline in older ages. This is a very good framework that holds true for many countries. However, there are also many countries to which it is not applicable. Notably, many countries in the African region have an age pattern similar to highly developed countries, according to estimates in the WHO report [2].

In 2012, the age curve peaked in the elderly in the majority of countries. There were more exceptions among females than males when genders were analysed separately. Most notably, there was a concentrated group of countries, including almost the whole Latin American region, where females in the age group 15–29 years had the highest suicide rate of all age groups (table 3). The list of such countries, however, was headed by India, where the suicide rate of females in the age group 15–29 years was estimated at 36.1 per 100,000, which was 2.2 times higher than the rate for the total population.

Another quite clear pattern was among females in age group 50–69 years. This age group had the highest suicide rate of all age groups in a number of Western European countries, particularly Northern Europe, as well as Canada and the USA. Within this set of countries, another clear distinction could be made. In continental Europe, the lowest suicide rate was among the age group 15–29 years, whereas in Northern Europe and North America the lowest suicide rate was among the oldest age group, which corresponds to the convex age pattern. The only exception was Sweden, where the pattern was similar to continental Europe (table 3).

This pattern where suicide risks among the elderly were somewhat lower in countries with higher economic development, although less pronounced, could also be found among males.

Table 3. Countries where female age groups 15–29 and 50–69 years had the highest suicide rate of all age groups per 100,000 of population in 2012

Country	Part of the world	All ages	Age groups				M/F ratio age group 15–29	M/F ratio age group 50–69
			15–29	30–49	50–69	70+		
India	Asia S	16.7	36.1	17.2	11.1	11.2	1.0	
Bolivia	America S Latin	8.6	17.2	7.7	5.5	8.6	1.4	
Kazakhstan	Asia C	9.4	15.0	10.5	9.5	11.9	3.1	
Turkmenistan	Asia C	7.5	12.0	8.0	9.4	12.0	3.3	
Ecuador	America S Latin	5.3	10.9	4.0	4.4	9.4	1.9	
El Salvador	America C Latin	5.8	9.6	5.9	6.5	6.9	2.7	
Guatemala	America C Latin	4.1	8.4	4.5	3.3	4.9	2.0	
Nicaragua	America C Latin	4.8	8.1	5.5	4.8	5.5	2.3	
Chile	America S Latin	6.0	8.0	7.9	6.9	5.0	3.1	
New Zealand	Oceania	5.4	7.3	7.1	5.5	5.5	2.5	
Mauritius	Africa	3.0	4.5	3.0	3.4	2.8	3.7	
Peru	America S Latin	2.1	4.0	1.9	2.0	3.1	1.5	
Colombia	America S Latin	1.9	3.6	1.6	2.2	0.4	3.4	
Costa Rica	America C Latin	2.2	3.2	3.2	2.5	0.6	3.8	
Mexico	America N Latin	1.7	3.1	2.0	1.3	0.5	2.9	
Panama	America C Latin	1.3	3.0	0.4	2.0	0.9	2.8	
Cyprus	Europe S	1.6	2.4	2.0	1.5	1.5	3.8	
Philippines	Asia SE	1.1	2.2	1.3	1.0	1.9	2.9	
Malta	Europe S	0.7	2.1	0.0	1.2	0.0	2.8	
Kuwait	Asia Arab	0.9	1.4	1.3	0.3	0.0	0.9	
Belize	America C	0.6	1.2	0.8	0.0	0.0	1.6	
Iceland	Europe N	7.5	4.5	9.8	17.1	2.5		1.7
Belgium	Europe W	9.7	4.9	11.1	16.4	12.4		2.0
Slovenia	Europe E	6.8	1.5	4.4	14.0	11.1		2.8
Cuba	America Carib.	6.0	1.5	4.2	13.4	12.0		2.7
France	Europe W	7.9	3.2	8.8	13.0	12.7		2.6
Sweden	Europe N	7.1	5.3	8.2	12.1	6.8		2.5
Switzerland	Europe W	6.6	4.4	5.9	11.7	8.8		2.4
Finland	Europe N	8.1	10.7	10.0	10.9	5.6		2.9
Denmark	Europe W	5.5	2.9	5.1	9.8	8.4		2.7
Moldova	Europe E	5.5	3.5	4.8	9.7	8.0		5.4
USA	America N	5.8	4.7	8.0	9.2	4.0		3.4
Norway	Europe N	5.8	5.5	7.6	8.6	5.2		2.4
Netherlands	Europe W	5.9	3.6	7.9	8.4	7.4		2.5
Ireland	Europe N	5.5	6.2	7.4	8.3	3.4		2.7
Canada	America N	5.5	5.2	7.1	8.0	3.3		2.9
Slovakia	Europe E	3.2	1.7	3.0	5.5	5.4		7.2
Israel	Asia W	2.4	1.8	3.3	5.0	3.4		3.7
Brazil	America S Latin	2.6	2.6	3.7	3.8	3.3		3.3

Carib. = Caribbean (for other abbreviations, see table 1 footnote).

Age and gender patterns of suicide demonstrate remarkable cross-cultural and historical stability [20, 21]. However, when significant variation or change can be observed, it is always worthwhile to investigate potential underlying triggers. Pampel [22] stated that age patterns of suicide become increasingly important as indicators of economic and social well-being.

Suicide Methods

According to the current diagnostic tool – ICD-10 – deaths from external causes are diagnosed in chapter XX under codes V1–Y98, with suicide as a separate subcategory under codes X60–X84. It includes codes for poisoning, hanging, drowning, firearm use, jumping, and others. Notably, the list of diagnoses is exactly the same for deaths of undetermined intent (Y10–Y34 in ICD-10), the only difference being whether the intent to die was uncertain. The list of diagnoses is also quite similar for homicides (X85–Y09 in ICD-10), the difference being auto-aggression in the case of suicides.

Data about methods are very informative but due to insufficient reporting the worldwide picture is not complete. Nevertheless, considerable variability can be found among developed countries where reporting is not deficient. According to the WHO report [2] in 2012, hanging accounts for 50% of suicides and firearms are the second most common method, accounting for 18% of suicides, which was driven by the USA, where firearms accounted for half of all suicides. A systematic review by Gunnell et al. [16] estimated that pesticide self-poisoning accounts for 30% of suicides globally. These deaths occur mostly in economically less developed countries.

Suicide Attempts

The WHO estimates that for each adult suicide there may have been more than 20 suicide attempts [2]. Suicide risk is much higher in individuals who previously made a suicide attempt and research shows that suicide attempt is the single most important predictor of death by suicide.

There are very few registries worldwide on suicide attempts. Most of those surveys are hospital based or rely on self-reports. Only a few surveys are administered to the same population over time. Comparisons between countries of self-reported suicide attempt rates are problematic, as the willingness to report suicidal behaviour varies by age, gender, ethnicity, religion, and other factors. Similarly to the suicide rates, the ratio of suicide attempt to suicide death shows wide variations by region, gender, age, and method of suicide.

Longitudinal epidemiological surveillance of both attempted and completed suicide on the population level, as well as samples collected in health care institutions, is of vital importance for planning and performing suicide preventive activities.

Suicide Prevention

The strong taboo surrounding suicide still exists and suicidal acts are associated with shame, uneasiness and guilt. As a result, suicides are concealed and the view that suicide is impossible to prevent or treat still prevails. These perceptions must be combatted by information underscoring the fact that suicide is preventable. However, different groups of suicidal persons require different strategies [23, 24].

In suicide prevention work, strategies can be directed to the health care services or at the general population. The health care approach is characterized by identifying risk groups, improving the diagnosis and treatment of suicidal patients and offering rehabilitation for suicide attempters. There are many pharmacological, psychotherapeutic and psychosocial treatments showing efficacy in the treatment and rehabilitation of suicidal persons [25].

The public health approach is directed at the general population. At the population level, restricting access to lethal means of suicide, developing policies to reduce the harmful use of alcohol and encouraging the media to follow responsible reporting practices on suicide are the most applied strategies to date. Preventive intervention for vulnerable populations and support for bereaved families and significant others who have lost a loved one by suicide are increasingly getting attention.

There is also a great need for preventive strategies for young people, as suicidal behaviours, according to the WHO global suicide report, constitute a great problem in young populations. An evidence-based method was developed in the EU-funded project 'Saving and Empowering Young Lives in Europe' (SEYLE) in 10 European countries. Results from the SEYLE cluster-randomized controlled trial demonstrated that the YAM (Youth Aware of Mental Health) programme (www.y-a-m.org), which is a universal school-based intervention, led to a significant reduction of incident suicide attempts and severe suicidal ideation with plans compared with the control group [26].

References

1 Durkheim E: Suicide: A Study in Sociology (1897). London/New York, Routledge Classics, 2002.
2 World Health Organization. Preventing Suicide: A Global Imperative. Geneva, World Health Organization, 2014.
3 Bertolote JM, Fleischmann A: Suicide and psychiatric diagnosis: A worldwide perspective. World Psychiatry 2002;1:181–185.
4 Värnik P: Suicide in the world. Int J Environ Res Public Health 2012;9:760–771.
5 Ajdacic-Gross V, Bopp M, Gostynski M, Lauber C, Gutzwiller F, Rössler W: Age-period-cohort analysis of Swiss suicide data, 1881–2000. Eur Arch Psychiatry Clin Neurosci 2006;256:207–214.
6 Ratnayeke L: Suicide in Sri Lanka; in Kosky RJ, Eshkevari HS, Goldney RD, Hassan RE (eds): Suicide Prevention: The Global Context. New York, Plenum Press, 1998, pp 139–142.
7 Shields LB, Hunsaker DM, Hunsaker JC III: Trends of suicide in the United States during the 20th century; in Tsokos M (ed): Forensic Pathology Reviews. Totowa, Humana Press, 2005, pp 305–335.
8 Jukkala T, Mäkinen IH, Stickley A: The historical development of suicide mortality in Russia, 1870–2007. Arch Suicide Res 2015;19:117–130.
9 Thomas K, Gunnell D: Suicide in England and Wales 1861–2007: a time-trends analysis. Int J Epidemiol 2010;39:1464–1475.

10 Condorelli R: A Bayesian analysis of suicide data. Qual Quant 2013;47:1143–1161.
11 Paerregaard G: Suicide in Denmark: a statistical review for the past 150 years. Suicide Life Threat Behav 1980;10:150–156.
12 Kushner HI: Suicide, gender, and the fear of modernity in nineteenth-century medical and social thought. J Soc Hist 1993;26:461–490.
13 Mościcki EK: Gender differences in completed and attempted suicides. Ann Epidemiol 1994;4:152–158.
14 Värnik A, Kolves K, van der Feltz-Cornelis CM, Marusic A, Oskarsson H, Palmer A, Reisch T, Scheerder G, Arensman E, Aromaa E, Giupponi G, Gusmao R, Maxwell M, Pull C, Szekely A, Sola VP, Hegerl U: Suicide methods in Europe: a gender-specific analysis of countries participating in the 'European Alliance Against Depression'. J Epidemiol Community Health 2008;62:545–551.
15 Canetto SS, Sakinofsky I: The gender paradox in suicide. Suicide Life Threat Behav 1998;28:1–23.
16 Gunnell D, Eddleston M, Phillips MR, Konradsen F: The global distribution of fatal pesticide self-poisoning: systematic review. BMC Public Health 2007;7:357.
17 Ramstedt M: Alcohol and suicide in 14 European countries. Addiction 2001;96(suppl 1):59–75.
18 Wasserman D, Värnik A, Eklund G: Male suicides and alcohol consumption in the former USSR. Acta Psychiatr Scand 1994;89:306–313.
19 Möller-Leimkühler AM: Barriers to help-seeking by men: a review of sociocultural and clinical literature with particular reference to depression. J Affect Disord 2002;71:1–9.
20 Girard C: Age, gender, and suicide: a cross-national analysis. Am Sociol Rev 1993;54:553–574.
21 Mäkinen IH, Wasserman D: Suicide mortality among immigrant Finnish Swedes. Arch Suicide Res 2003;7:93–106.
22 Pampel FC: Cohort size and age-specific suicide rates: a contingent relationship. Demography 1996;33:341–355.
23 Wasserman D: Suicide: An Unnecessary Death. London, Martin Dunitz, 2001.
24 Wasserman D, Wasserman C: Oxford Textbook of Suicidology and Suicide Prevention. London, Oxford University Press, 2009.
25 Wasserman D, Rihmer Z, Rujescu D, Sarchiapone M, Sokolowski M, Titelman D, Zalsman G, Zemishlany Z, Carli V: The European Psychiatric Association (EPA) guidance on suicide treatment and prevention. Eur Psychiatry 2012;27:129–141.
26 Wasserman D, Hoven CW, Wasserman C, Wall M, Eisenberg R, Hadlaczky G, Kelleher I, Sarchiapone M, Apter A, Balazs J, Bobes J, Brunner R, Corcoran P, Cosman D, Guillemin F, Haring C, Iosue M, Kaess M, Kahn J-P, Keeley H, Musa GJ, Nemes B, Postuvan V, Saiz P, Reiter-Theil S, Varnik A, Varnik P, Carli V: School-based suicide prevention programmes: the SEYLE cluster-randomised, controlled trial. Lancet 2015;385:1536–1544.

Dr. Peeter Värnik
Estonian-Swedish Mental Health and Suicidology Institute (ERSI)
Õie 39
EE–11615 Tallinn (Estonia)
E-Mail peeterv@suicidology.ee

Kaschka WP, Rujescu D (eds): Biological Aspects of Suicidal Behavior.
Adv Biol Psychiatry. Basel, Karger, 2016, vol 30, pp 11–20 (DOI: 10.1159/000435767)

Suicidal Ideation, Suicide Attempts and Completed Suicide in Adolescents: Neurobiological Aspects

Marco Sarchiapone • Marianna D'Aulerio • Miriam Iosue

Department of Medicine and Health Sciences, University of Molise, Campobasso, Italy

Abstract

Suicidal behavior is a complex and multidetermined phenomenon that affects countries around the world and all age groups. Adolescence is a critical period in human growth, ranging from 10 to 19 years of age, and it is one of the stages of life with the highest risk for the adoption of risky and suicidal behavior. In the USA, for youths between the ages of 10 and 24 years, suicide is the third leading cause of death. Deaths from youth suicide are only part of the problem. Among the age group of 15–24 years, it is estimated that approximately 100–200 suicide attempts take place for every completed suicide. In recent years, several studies and research projects have been conducted to better understand teenage suicide in order to implement effective prevention strategies. However, the majority of these have focused on psychosocial aspects of suicidal behavior among young people, such that the neurobiological aspects associated with it still remain unclear to a large degree. However, the involvement of specific abnormalities in neurobiological mechanisms as predisposing to, or as risk factors for, suicidal behavior is supported by several research studies, which have found an association between young suicide and abnormalities in the hypothalamic-pituitary-adrenal axis, serotonergic system, signal transduction pathways, and inflammatory markers.

Adolescence is a critical period in human growth and development that occurs after childhood and before adulthood, ranging from 10 to 19 years of age. This is a crucial period for laying the foundations for healthy development and good mental health. In fact, during adolescence, which is characterized by a particular vulnerability to the pressures and challenges in daily lives, it is possible to adopt different health risk behaviors. These behaviors, which are established during adolescence and often maintained into adulthood, may affect mental health and well-being in later life [1]. Suicidal behavior is one of the extreme consequences of a psychological disease that is undetected and untreated.

Suicidal behavior represents a serious public health problem, since suicide is among the leading causes of death worldwide, especially among adolescents and young adults

[2]. In the USA, among youths aged 10–24 years, suicide is the third leading cause of death. The top three methods used in this age group include firearms (45%), suffocation (40%) and poisoning (8%) [3]. According to the WHO [1], suicidal thoughts and behaviors are increasing in Western countries, especially in Europe. Every year, in the 27 EU member states, approximately 63,000 Europeans die by suicide – one of the highest suicide rates in the world [4]. Among this population, the rate of suicide increases with age and is substantially higher in boys than in girls [5, 3]. Of the reported suicides in the age group of 10–24 years, 81% of the deaths were males and 19% were females. Girls, however, are more likely to report attempting suicide than boys [3].

The deaths from youth suicide are only part of the problem. Among the age group of 15–24 years, it is estimated that approximately 100–200 suicide attempts take place for every completed suicide [6].

The vast majority of youths with suicidal behaviors have preexisting mental disorders. Nock et al. [2] found that the vast majority of adolescents with a lifetime history of suicide ideation (89.3%) and attempt (96.1%) meet lifetime criteria for primary DSM-IV disorders and that most suicidal adolescents (>80%) receive some form of mental health treatment. In most cases (>55%), treatment starts prior to the onset of suicidal behaviors but fails to prevent these behaviors from occurring.

Despite extensive studies of psychosocial factors associated with youth suicide and suicidal behavior, the neurobiology of suicidal behavior still remains unclear to a large degree. However, several research studies have shown that specific abnormalities in neurobiological mechanisms may be associated with suicidal behavior, at least among adults [7, 8].

The Neurobiology of Suicidal Behavior

The studies of biological abnormalities associated with suicidal behavior – performed in biomaterials such as blood cells, cerebrospinal fluid (CSF) and plasma obtained from suicidal patients – have shed some light on this matter. The studies conducted on postmortem brain samples of suicide victims allow a better understanding of the pathomechanisms in the brain [9]. As a result, an involvement of serotonergic and noradrenergic systems, abnormalities in the hypothalamic-pituitary-adrenocortical axis, signal transduction pathways, and inflammatory markers (cytokines in the postmortem brain) were found in teenage suicide [10].

The Serotonergic System

Serotonergic (5-HT) dysfunction has been extensively studied in adults and has been postulated as a biological marker for suicide [11]. The studies that analyze this association include several elements such as serotonin receptors, serotonin transporter and tryptophan hydroxylase [9].

Several research studies have suggested a role of serotonin in suicide. The pioneer studies of Asberg et al. [12] and Linnoila and Virkkunen [13] found an association between a low CSF concentration of 5-hydroxyindoleacetic acid (5-HIAA) – the main metabolite of serotonin – and increased impulsiveness, impaired control of aggressive behaviors and suicide attempts [14]. Brent and Mann [15], in their postmortem and imaging studies of persons who had completed or attempted suicide, identified alterations in the number and function of serotonin receptors in the regions of the prefrontal cortex (PFC) that are involved in emotion regulation and behavioral inhibition.

Even if the correlation between suicidal behavior and the serotonergic system in adulthood is well analyzed, to date, few of these studies have been conducted on samples of adolescents [16].

Pandey et al. [17] analyzed the relationship between some abnormalities of serotonin (5-HT), the receptor subtypes – specifically the 5-HT_{2A} receptor – and suicidal behavior. In their study, the authors observed the 5-HT_{2A} receptor levels in the PFC, hippocampus and nucleus accumbens of postmortem brains obtained from 15 teenage suicide victims and 15 psychiatrically normal teenage subjects who died of other causes. The cellular localization of the 5-HT_{2A} receptors was determined by means of gold immunolabeling. The authors found that 5-HT_{2A} receptor binding sites, protein and mRNA expression were more numerous in the PFC and hippocampus of teenage suicide victims than in normal subjects. These brain regions are implicated in emotion, stress and cognition; similar results were also observed in adults who died by suicide. There was no higher level in the nucleus accumbens, which is implicated in drug dependence and craving. The findings of the authors suggest that a higher level of 5-HT_{2A} receptors may be one of the neurobiological abnormalities associated with teenage suicide.

Tyano et al. [18] studied the relationship of plasma serotonin (p5-HT) levels and psychometric measures between depressed suicidal adolescents and controls. The sample, composed of 211 Israeli adolescents, was divided into four groups (suicidal psychiatric inpatients, nonsuicidal psychiatric inpatients, adolescents referred to the emergency room due to a suicide attempt, and a community-based control group from 4 high schools in the same catchment areas). All adolescents were interviewed and assessed for violence, aggression, depression, impulsivity, anger, and anxiety. The results showed significantly lower levels of p5-HT in the control group compared with all other groups and a significant negative correlation between p5-HT level and suicidal behavior severity among the suicidal inpatients. There was no difference in serotonin levels among psychiatric diagnostic categories.

However, Picouto et al. [11], who conducted a comprehensive review on the role of serotonergic (5-HT) dysfunction in suicidal behavior – both in adults and adolescents – noticed that the studies on 5-HT conducted in adults and replicated in adolescents yielded inconsistent results. For this reason, they suggested that subsequent studies on the neurobiology of adolescent suicide should consider the biological specificities of this life stage and gender differences during this period in an effort to integrate findings in the psychological and biological domains.

The Hypothalamic-Pituitary-Adrenal Axis

Several studies have reported an association between abnormalities in the hypothalamic-pituitary-adrenal (HPA) axis and suicidal behaviors [19].

Stress plays a major role in the various pathophysiological processes associated with mood disorders and suicidal behavior [20]. Moreover, high stress levels may cause unfavorable effects in different brain functions such as those of the HPA axis. Indeed, the HPA axis is responsible for the modulation of cortisol levels – one of the main stress hormones.

Pandey et al. [21] analyzed the protein and gene expression of glucocorticoid and mineralocorticoid receptors in the PFC, hippocampus, subiculum, and amygdala in a sample of 48 teenagers (24 suicide victims and 24 control subjects). The aim of the study was to test the hypothesis that the reported dysregulation of the HPA axis in suicide may be related to a disturbed feedback inhibition caused by decreased corticoid receptors in the brain. The results showed a significant decrease both in the protein and gene expression of glucocorticoid-α in the PFC and amygdala, but not in the hippocampus or subiculum, and in the mRNA levels of glucocorticoid-inducible target gene GILZ in the PFC and amygdaloid nuclei of teenage suicide victims but not in the control group. In contrast, no differences were found both in the protein and gene expression of mineralocorticoid receptors in any of the studied areas and the expression of glucocorticoid-β in the PFC between teenage suicide victims and normal control subjects.

Abnormal HPA axis functioning associated with an anomalous interaction with other systems such as the serotonergic system may be one of the neurobiological correlates of emotion dysregulation, with important implications for the adolescent. Indeed, psychopathological conditions such as depression or childhood psychological trauma increase suicidal risk in adolescents and are also associated with HPA axis dysregulation. Moreover, emotion dysregulation could be a predisposing factor that augments the vulnerability to suffer from psychiatric conditions [22].

Signal Transduction Studies in Teenage Suicide

Studies conducted on the involvement of the abnormalities of the serotonergic mechanism in suicidal behavior have allowed us to expand our knowledge on the neurobiology of suicidal behavior. The presence of abnormalities in specific serotonin receptor subtypes such as the 5-HT_{2A} receptor, which is linked to signal transduction pathways in the brains of suicide victims, has motivated an increase in studies on the role of transduction processes in the understanding of the biological aspects of suicide [23]. To date, most studies have focused their attention on the abnormalities in the component of this signaling system, indicating a role of abnormalities of phosphoinositide (PI), adenylyl cyclase, MAP kinase, and brain-derived neurotrophic factor (BDNF) signaling systems [24].

Protein Kinase A

Protein kinase A (PKA), also known as cyclic AMP (cAMP)-dependent protein kinase, is a family of enzymes whose activity is dependent on cellular levels of cAMP. PKA has several functions in the cell. It is involved in regulating gene transcription, cell survival and plasticity [11] and is implicated in the pathophysiology of depression and suicide [25]. While analyzing PKA and protein kinase C (PKC) protein levels in human postmortem brain tissue in a sample of 20 persons with major depression and 20 controls, Shelton et al. [26] found that the group with major depression, and in particular those who died by suicide, had low PKA RIα (regulatory Iα) and PKA Cα (catalytic α), supporting the role of abnormalities of these two key kinases in the physiopathology of suicide and mental illness.

In a postmortem brain study, Pandey et al. [27] analyzed the PKA activity and the protein and mRNA expression of different subunits of PKA in cytosol and membrane of the PFC, hippocampus and nucleus accumbens of 17 teenage suicide victims and 17 nonpsychiatric control subjects. The authors found that in the group of teenage suicide victims PKA activity was significantly decreased in the PFC but not in the hippocampus. Moreover, the protein expression of two PKA subunits, PKA RIα and PKA RIβ, were significantly decreased in both membrane and cytosol fractions of the PFC and in the nucleus accumbens of teenage suicide victims compared with controls.

Further studies showed significant differences between teenage and adult suicide victims. Decreased cAMP binding and PKA activity was found in both teenage and adult suicide victims. However, in teenagers, abnormalities of RIα and RIβ subunits seem to be involved, while decreased RIIα and Cβ were found in adults. Considering these conflicting results, more studies are needed to better understand the implications of these observations with regard to the pathophysiology of teenage and adult suicides.

Protein Kinase C

Protein kinase C (PKC) is a critical phosphorylating enzyme in the PI signaling pathway. It is present in various tissues, including the brain, and is localized presynaptically and postsynaptically. PKC is involved in the pathogenesis of mood disorders and is a target for the therapeutic action of mood-stabilizing drugs [28].

Despite the discovery of the implication of PKC in the pathogenesis of mental disorders and suicidal behavior, very few studies have been conducted to verify this relationship in adolescents and, to date, it seems that only a couple of studies have been conducted to examine this relationship.

One of these research studies analyzed the relationship between abnormalities in PKC and suicidal behavior using postmortem brain materials pertaining to 17 teenage suicide victims and 17 nonpsychiatric control subjects. The authors reported a statistically significant decrease in PKC in membrane and cytosol fractions of the PFC and hippocampus of teenage suicide victims. Statistically significant decreases in protein levels of PKC-α, -βI, -βII, and -γ isozymes were also observed in both of these fractions. These decreases were associated with decreases in levels of their respective messenger RNAs. The authors suggest that the pathogenesis of teenage suicide may be associated with abnormalities in PKC and that PKC may be a target for therapeutic intervention in patients with suicidal behavior, since many physiological functions are mediated through phosphorylation by PKC and because PKC is a target for the therapeutic action of psychoactive drugs [28].

Phospholipase C in Suicide

The enzyme PI-specific phospholipase C (PI-PLC) is a component of the PI signal transduction system and some studies have shown its implication in neuropsychiatric disorders, including suicidal behavior in the young and adults [29, 30]. Lo Vasco et al. [29] reported a reduction of overall PLC expression and a complex reorganization of the isoforms in postmortem brain samples of 28 individuals who committed suicide compared with controls.

Concerning adolescents, a study conducted on the postmortem brains of 18 teenage suicide subjects and 18 matched comparison subjects showed that PI-PLC activity and immunolabeling of the specific PLC-β1 isozyme, in both membrane and cytosol fractions of Brodmann areas 8 and 9 combined, were significantly lower among suicides than among controls. Moreover, in the group of teenage suicide subjects, a significant correlation between PI-PLC activity and protein levels of the PLC-β1 isozyme was identified. These results supported the role of PLC in the pathophysiology of suicidal behavior [30].

Transcription Factor CREB

The cAMP response element binding protein (CREB) is a transcription factor activated by PKA and PKC that phosphorylates several transcription factors, which then influence gene expression.

The literature indicates an implication of CREB in the pathophysiology of suicide [9]. A significant increase in the levels of CREB, both in total and phosphorylated form, was found in the brains of depressed suicide victims compared with those of control subjects. The increases in CREB were specifically observed in antidepressant-free subjects but not in the antidepressant-treated subjects, suggesting the role of the cAMP signaling system in the therapy with antidepressants [31]. The research conducted by Young et al. [32] reported increased numbers of phosphorylated CREB-stained cells in several amygdalar nuclei in subjects who had died by suicide. In contrast, patients treated with lithium at the time of death had significantly lower phosphorylated CREB levels in the same region. However, the association between the increase in CREB and suicide was not confirmed in a study by Dwivedi et al. [33], which reported a significant reduction of the protein expression of CREB in the nuclear fractions of both the PFC and the hippocampus obtained from suicide victims compared with control subjects. Also, Pandey et al. [34] reported a specific decrease in CRE-DNA binding and mRNA as well as the protein expression of CREB in the PFC of teenage suicide victims. However, they did not find any significant differences in hippocampal CREB levels between teenage suicides and controls.

Brain-Derived Neurotrophic Factor and Tyrosine Kinase B Receptors in Suicide

BDNF is the most abundant neurotrophin in the brain. Even if its role in the pathophysiology of anxiety and depression is clear, less is known about its role in suicidal behavior. In fact, BDNF is involved in the pathophysiology of many psychiatric disorders associated with suicidal behavior and its dysregulation could be associated with increased suicidality, independent of psychiatric diagnoses [35]. Keller et al., in their study conducted in 2010, reported a decrease of BDNF levels in the brain and plasma of suicide subjects; in fact, a statistically significant increase of DNA methylation was found in the Wernicke area at specific CpG sites in BDNF promoter/exon IV compared with nonsuicide control subjects [36]. Also, Dwivedi et al. [37], analyzing Brodmann area 9 and the hippocampus of 27 suicide subjects and 21 nonpsychiatric control subjects, found that the BDNF and tyrosine kinase B (TrkB) were significantly reduced in both the PFC and hippocampus in suicide subjects compared with those in control subjects.

BDNF is involved in the regulation and growth of neurons during childhood and adolescence. For example, it is hypnotized that the serotonin dysfunctions associated with adolescent and adult suicidal behavior could be related to the low level of BDNF, which impedes the normal development of serotonin neurons during brain development. This dysfunction could play a more significant role in the pathophysiology of psychiatric disorders and suicidal behavior in adolescents than in adults [35]. Using the Western blot technique, the protein expression of BDNF was determined in the PFC, Brodmann area 9 and hippocampus in a sample of 29 teenage suicide victims and 25 matched normal control subjects. The results showed a decrease in the protein expression of BDNF in the PFC of teenage suicide victims compared with normal control subjects but no change in the hippocampus. Also, the protein expression of TrkB full-length receptors was significantly decreased in both the PFC and hippocampus of teenage suicide victims. The mRNA expression of both BDNF and TrkB was significantly decreased in the PFC and hippocampus of teenage suicide victims compared with normal control subjects. All these data suggest that altered BDNF may represent a major vulnerability factor in teenage suicidal behavior [38].

Cytokines and Suicidal Behavior

The association of cytokines with the pathophysiology of depression, psychiatric disorders and suicidal behavior is well described and documented. Significantly higher levels of cytokine were found in blood, CSF and postmortem brain samples of patients with suicidality. The levels of interleukin (IL)-1β and IL-6 were most robustly associated with suicidality and these cytokines may help distinguish suicidal from nonsuicidal patients [39]. IL-6 is significantly higher in the CSF in suicide attempters, possibly through mechanisms involving alterations of dopamine and serotonin metabolism [40]. Ducasse et al. [41] conducted the first meta-analysis of studies comparing the plasma and CSF concentrations of cytokines in suicidal patients with those of nonsuicidal patients or healthy controls. The meta-analysis comprised a total sample of 494 suicidal patients, 497 nonsuicidal patients and 398 healthy controls. The results obtained supported the hypothesis of altered inflammatory markers in suicidal patients for both proinflammatory (IL-2) and anti-inflammatory (IL-4 and TGF-β) cytokines. In a study conducted in 2012, Pandey et al. [27] measured the gene and protein expression levels of proinflammatory cytokines IL-1β, IL-6 and tissue necrosis factor (TNF)-α in the PFC of 24 teenage suicide victims and 24 matched normal control subjects. Their results confirmed the role of cytokines also in adolescent suicide – the mRNA and protein expression levels of IL-1β, IL-6 and TNF-α were significantly increased in Brodmann area 10 of the suicide victims, suggesting an important role for IL-1β, IL-6 and TNF-α in the pathophysiology of suicidal behavior.

Conclusion

Suicide among adolescents is a serious problem that the world cannot underestimate. For this reason it is necessary to improve the studies and research regarding the risk factors for suicide in order to identify and properly treat the adolescents at risk. The studies on suicidal behavior in adolescents correlate with several neurobiological evidence, independent of underlying psychiatric disorders. These include, for example, the involvement of the HPA axis [42], serotonergic system, signal transduction pathways and inflammatory markers. Even if, in recent years, much has been done with respect to the psychosocial aspects of suicide, much remains to be done with regard to understanding the neurobiological aspects of suicidal behavior. Moreover, most of these studies were conducted on samples of adult subjects, while recent research studies suggest that suicidal behavior in teenagers can have both common and different neurobiological abnormalities compared with adult suicide [23].

References

1 WHO: Documents on adolescent health. http://www.who.int/maternal_child_adolescent/documents/adolescent/en/ (accessed May 3, 2015).

2 Nock MK, Green JG, Hwang I, McLaughlin KA, Sampson NA, Zaslavsky AM, Kessler RC: Prevalence, correlates and treatment of lifetime suicidal behavior among adolescents: results from the National Comorbidity Survey Replication – Adolescent Supplement (NCS-A). JAMA Psychiatry 2013;70:300–310.

3 Centers for Disease Control and Prevention. http://www.cdc.gov/ (accessed April 27, 2015).

4 Eurostat: Eurostat Year Book 2009. http://epp.eurostat.ec.europa.eu/portal/page/portal/publications/eurostat_yearbook.

5 Bridge JA, Goldstein TR, Brent DA: Adolescent suicide and suicidal behavior. J Child Psychol Psychiatry 2006;47:372–394.

6 Bertolote JM, Fleischmann A, De Leo D, Phillips MR, Botega NJ, Vijayakumar L, Wasserman D: Repetition of suicide attempts: data from emergency care settings in five culturally different low- and middle-income countries participating in the WHO SUPRE-MISS Study. Crisis 2010;31:194–201.

7 Mann JJ: The neurobiology of suicide. Nat Med 1998;4:25–30.

8 Underwood MD, Mann JJ, Arango V: Serotonergic and noradrenergic neurobiology of alcoholic suicide. Alcohol Clin Exp Res 2004;28(5 suppl):57S–69S.

9 Furczyk K, Schutová B, Michel TM, Thome J, Büttner A: The neurobiology of suicide – a review of post-mortem studies. J Mol Psychiatry 2013;1:2.

10 Dwivedi Y, Pandey GN: Elucidating biological risk factors in suicide: role of protein kinase A. Prog Neuropsychopharmacol Biol Psychiatry 2011;35:831–841.

11 Picouto MD, Villar F, Braquehais MD: The role of serotonin in adolescent suicide: theoretical, methodological, and clinical concerns. Int J Adolesc Med Health 2015;27:129–133.

12 Asberg M, Träskman L, Thorén P: 5-HIAA in the cerebrospinal fluid. A biochemical suicide predictor? Arch Gen Psychiatry 1976;33:1193–1197.

13 Linnoila VM, Virkkunen M: Aggression, suicidality, and serotonin. J Clin Psychiatry 1992;53(suppl):46–51.

14 Perroud N, Salzmann A, Saiz PA, Baca-Garcia E, Sarchiapone M, Garcia-Portilla, MP; European Research Consortium for Suicide (EURECA): Rare genotype combination of the serotonin transporter gene associated with treatment response in severe personality disorder. Am J Med Genet B Neuropsychiatr Genet 2010;153B:1494–1497.

15 Brent DA, Mann JJ: Familial pathways to suicidal behavior – understanding and preventing suicide among adolescents. N Engl J Med 2006;355:2719–2721.

16 Mann JJ: Neurobiology of suicidal behaviour. Nat Rev Neurosci 2003;4:819–828.

17 Pandey GN, Dwivedi Y, Rizavi HS, Ren X, Pandey SC, Pesold C, Tamminga CA: Higher expression of serotonin 5-HT_{2A} receptors in the postmortem brains of teenage suicide victims. Am J Psychiatry 2002;159:419–429.

18 Tyano S, Zalsman G, Ofek H, Blum I, Apter A, Wolovik L, Weizman A: Plasma serotonin levels and suicidal behavior in adolescents. Eur Neuropsychopharmacol 2006;16:49–57.

19 Wasserman D, Wasserman J, Sokolowski M: Genetics of HPA-axis, depression and suicidality. Eur Psychiatry 2010;25:278–280.

20 Sarchiapone M, D'Aulerio M: Genetic risk factors for suicidal behavior; in Cannon KE, Hudzik TJ (eds): Suicide: Phenomenology and Neurobiology. New York, Springer, 2014, pp 125–140.

21 Pandey GN, Rizavi HS, Ren X, Dwivedi Y, Palkovits M: Region-specific alterations in glucocorticoid receptor expression in the postmortem brain of teenage suicide victims. Psychoneuroendocrinology 2013;38:2628–2639.

22 Braquehais MD, Picouto MD, Casas M, Sher L: Hypothalamic-pituitary-adrenal axis dysfunction as a neurobiological correlate of emotion dysregulation in adolescent suicide. World J Pediatr 2012;8:197–206.

23 Pandey GN: Signal transduction abnormalities in suicide: focus on phosphoinositide signaling system. CNS Neurol Disord Drug Targets 2013;12:941–953.

24 Pandey GN, Dwivedi Y: Neurobiology of teenage suicide; in Dwivedi Y (ed): The Neurobiological Basis of Suicide. Boca Raton, CRC Press, 2012.

25 Pandey GN, Dwivedi Y, Ren X, Rizavi HS, Mondal AC, Shukla PK, Conley RR: Brain region specific alterations in the protein and mrna levels of protein kinase a subunits in the post-mortem brain of teenage suicide victims. Neuropsychopharmacology 2005;30:1548–1556.

26 Shelton RC, Hal Manier D, Lewis DA: Protein kinases A and C in post-mortem prefrontal cortex from persons with major depression and normal controls. Int J Neuropsychopharmacol 2009;12: 1223–1232.

27 Pandey GN, Rizavi HS, Ren X, Fareed J, Hoppensteadt DA, Roberts RC, Dwivedi Y: Proinflammatory cytokines in the prefrontal cortex of teenage suicide victims. J Psychiatr Res 2012;46: 57–63.

28 Pandey GN, Dwivedi Y, Rizavi HS, Ren X, Conley RR: Decreased catalytic activity and expression of protein kinase C isozymes in teenage suicide victims: a postmortem brain study. Arch Gen Psychiatry 2004;61:685–693.

29 Lo Vasco VR, Leopizzi M, Della Rocca C, Fais P, Montisci M, Cecchetto G: Impairment and reorganization of the phosphoinositide-specific phospholipase C enzymes in suicide brains. J Affect Disord 2015;174:324–328.

30 Pandey GN, Dwivedi Y, Pandey SC, Teas SS, Conley RR, Roberts RC, Tamminga CA: Low phosphoinositide-specific phospholipase C activity and expression of phospholipase C β1 protein in the prefrontal cortex of teenage suicide subjects. Am J Psychiatry 1999; 156:1895–1901.

31 Odagaki Y, García-Sevilla JA, Huguelet P, La Harpe R, Koyama T, Guimón J: Cyclic AMP-mediated signaling components are upregulated in the prefrontal cortex of depressed suicide victims. Brain Res 2001; 898:224–231.

32 Young LT, Bezchlibnyk YB, Chen B, Wang J-F, MacQueen GM: Amygdala cyclic adenosine monophosphate response element binding protein phosphorylation in patients with mood disorders: effects of diagnosis, suicide, and drug treatment. Biol Psychiatry 2004;55:570–577.

33 Dwivedi Y, Rao JS, Rizavi HS, Kotowski J, Conley RR, Roberts RC, Pandey GN: Abnormal expression and functional characteristics of cyclic adenosine monophosphate response element binding protein in postmortem brain of suicide subjects. Arch Gen Psychiatry 2003;60:273–282.

34 Pandey GN, Dwivedi Y, Ren X, Rizavi HS, Roberts RC, Conley RR: Cyclic AMP response element-binding protein in post-mortem brain of teenage suicide victims: specific decrease in the prefrontal cortex but not the hippocampus. Int J Neuropsychopharmacol 2007;10:621–629.

35 Sher L: The role of brain-derived neurotrophic factor in the pathophysiology of adolescent suicidal behavior. Int J Adolesc Med Health 2011;23:181–185.

36 Keller S, Sarchiapone M, Zarrilli F, et al: Increased BDNF promoter methylation in the Wernicke area of suicide subjects. Arch Gen Psychiatry 2010;67: 258–267.

37 Dwivedi Y, Rizavi HS, Conley RR, Roberts RC, Tamminga CA, Pandey GN: Altered gene expression of brain-derived neurotrophic factor and receptor tyrosine kinase B in postmortem brain of suicide subjects. Arch Gen Psychiatry 2003;60:804–815.

38 Pandey GN, Ren X, Rizavi HS, Conley RR, Roberts RC, Dwivedi Y: Brain-derived neurotrophic factor and tyrosine kinase B receptor signalling in postmortem brain of teenage suicide victims. Int J Neuropsychopharmacol 2008;11:1047–1061.

39 Black C, Miller BJ: Meta-analysis of cytokines and chemokines in suicidality: distinguishing suicidal versus nonsuicidal patients. Biol Psychiatry 2015;78: 28–37.

40 Lindqvist D, Janelidze S, Hagell P, Erhardt S, Samuelsson M, Minthon L, Brundin L: Interleukin-6 is elevated in the cerebrospinal fluid of suicide attempters and related to symptom severity. Biol Psychiatry 2009;66:287–292.

41 Ducasse D, Olié E, Guillaume S, Artéro S, Courtet P: A meta-analysis of cytokines in suicidal behavior. Brain Behav Immun 2015;46:203–211.

42 Zalsman G: Genetics of suicidal behavior in children and adolescents; in Dwivedi Y (ed): The Neurobiological Basis of Suicide. Boca Raton, CRC Press, 2012.

Marco Sarchiapone
Department of Medicine and Health Sciences, University of Molise
Via Francesco de Sanctis 1
IT–86100 Campobasso (Italy)
E-Mail marco.sarchiapone@me.com

Kaschka WP, Rujescu D (eds): Biological Aspects of Suicidal Behavior.
Adv Biol Psychiatry. Basel, Karger, 2016, vol 30, pp 21–36 (DOI: 10.1159/000435768)

Serotonergic and Noradrenergic Neurotransmitter Systems in Suicide

Yogesh Dwivedi

Department of Psychiatry and Behavioral Neurobiology, University of Alabama at Birmingham, Birmingham, Ala., USA

Abstract

Suicide is a major public concern. About one million people commit suicide every year worldwide. In the teenage population, it is the third leading cause of death in the USA. Although the underlying pathophysiology of suicide is not very well understood, postmortem brain studies have provided a greater understanding of the neurobiological abnormalities associated with suicide. This chapter discusses the role of neurotransmitter systems, particularly the serotonergic and noradrenergic systems, in suicidal behavior. Since these neurotransmitters mediate their functional responses by activating intracellular signaling pathways, a detailed account of changes in receptor signaling has been discussed. Major emphasis has been given to the phosphoinositide and adenylyl cyclase-cyclic adenosine monophosphate signaling pathways as these signaling components have been shown to be activated by both the serotonergic and noradrenergic pathways. More specifically, the role of GTP binding proteins and downstream effector molecules protein kinase C and protein kinase A and the regulation of target gene brain-derived neurotrophic factor have been discussed. Altogether, these studies provide a comprehensive knowledge of neurobiological abnormalities associated with suicide and provide vulnerability factors that may predispose a person to suicidal behavior.

In the past two decades, there are multiple lines of evidence that point to a role of biological factors in the etiology and pathophysiology of suicide. Most of these biological factors are associated with abnormal stress response and impulsive aggressive behavior. Because of the critical role played by the serotonergic system in impulsive aggressive behavior, the serotonergic system has been the most extensively studied neurotransmitter system in suicide. Although comparatively less studied, the central noradrenergic system, which plays key roles in stress response, attention, memory, sleep-wake cycle, decision making, and regulation of sympathetic states, has also shown a strong correlation with suicidal behavior. Intracellular signaling systems mediated by the binding of neurotransmitters to receptors facilitate behavioral and environmental adaptations, which are primarily mediated through the regulation of neural plasticity and the integration of physiological processes. Each signaling pathway has multiple levels of controlling mechanisms and components of various signaling pathways interact with each other to integrate the functional response. The present chapter will elaborate on the role of the serotonergic and noradrenergic systems in suicide based on findings in the human postmortem brain. In addition, the role of intracellular signaling pathways, particularly phosphoinositide (PI) and adenylyl cyclase-cyclic adenosine monophosphate (cAMP) signaling, in the context of suicidal behavior will be discussed. The genetic aspects of these neurotransmitter systems in suicide have been discussed in other chapters.

Serotonergic System in Suicide

5-Hydroxyindoleacetic Acid and Serotonin Transporter in Suicide

5-Hydroxyindoleacetic acid (5-HIAA) is the main metabolite of serotonin. Recently, Bach et al. [1] examined levels of 5-HT and 5-HIAA in the brainstem of suicide victims and found that the levels of both 5-HT and 5-HIAA are significantly increased throughout the rostrocaudal extent of the brainstem dorsal raphe nucleus (DRN) and median raphe nucleus (MRN). The extracellular levels of 5-HT or uptake of 5-HT are regulated by the serotonin transporter 5-HTT, both in central and peripheral systems [2]. A large number of studies have been done in platelets of suicidal patients, which indicate that serotonin uptake and 5-HTT levels are decreased in suicidal patients [3, 4]. In the central serotonergic system, 5-HTT is localized on the terminals of 5-HT neurons. Using ^{3}H-imipramine as ligand, several studies have shown lower 5-HTT in postmortem brains of suicide subjects [for review, see 5]. Using ^{3}H-cyanoimipramine, receptor autoradiography studies by Arango et al. [6, 7] showed reduced 5-HTT binding in the ventral prefrontal cortex (PFC) of depressed suicides. Similar changes were reported by Austin and O'Donnell [8], who found a deficit in the length and density of 5-HTT-immunoreactive neurons. Arango et al. [9] also noted that although there was no change in total 5-HTT mRNA in the brainstem, depressed suicides had fewer 5-HTT-expressing neurons and these neurons had higher 5-HTT transcriptional capacity. Recently, Okada et al. [10] examined DNA methylation profiles at the CpG island of SLC6A4 as a diagnostic biomarker for major depression. Although they did not find differences in methylation between depressed and healthy controls, they did, however, find that the methylation rates for several CpGs differed significantly after antidepressant treatment. These results suggest that a pretreatment methylation rate of SLC6A4 is associated with therapeutic responses to antidepressants in unmedicated patients with major depression.

Serotonin Receptors in Suicide

Serotonin receptors have been classified into several families and subtypes. Of these, 5-HT_{1A} and 5-HT_{2A} receptors have been the most implicated in suicidal behavior. In addition, some reports also show the involvement of 5-HT_{2C} receptors in suicide.

5-HT_{1A} Receptors

5-HT_{1A} receptors are expressed both pre- and postsynaptically. In the DRN, the 5-HT_{1A} receptor functions as a somatodendritic inhibitory autoreceptor on 5-HT neurons [11]. Greater autoinhibition of the 5-HT_{1A} receptor in the brainstem raphe nuclei may be a mechanism that contributes to reduced serotonergic neurotransmission in the PFC of suicide subjects [12]. Autoradiography studies of Brodmann's areas 45 and 46 using ^{3}H-8OH-DPAT show a significant increase in the ventrolateral PFC of suicide victims compared with control subjects. However, no changes were found in Brodmann's areas 8, 9, 11, 12, 24, or 32 of suicide victims [6]. 5-HT_{1A} autoreceptor levels have been shown to be elevated in the midbrain of suicide subjects by some [12], but not all [9], investigators. The apparent discrepancy between these findings could be associated with the brain regions examined. Whereas Stockmeier et al. [12] examined the most rostral part of the DRN, an increase in 5-HT_{1A} receptors in the rostral part of the DRN in suicides and a decrease in the remaining part of the DRN could result in a net decrease in binding in the DRN [13]. 5-HT_{1A} receptors have also been studied in the hippocampus of suicide victims. Joyce et al. [14] found an increase in 5-HT_{1A} receptor binding sites in the CA1 area of the hippocampus of suicide victims. However, studies by Stockmeier et al. [15] and Dillon et al. [16] did not show any difference. Recently, Sullivan et al. [17] determined the relationships between brain 5-HT_{1A} binding and subjects with suicidal behavior major depressive disorder (MDD) using PET and the 5-HT_{1A} antagonist radiotracer ^{11}C-labeled WAY 100635. They found that raphe nuclei 5-HT_{1A} binding potential was 45% greater in higher-lethality attempters compared with lower-lethality attempters, whereas no difference was observed in the PFC regions. 5-HT_{1A} binding potential in the raphe nuclei of suicide attempters was positively correlated with the lethality rating and the subjective lethal intent factor based on the most recent suicide attempt. Suicide ideation in participants with MDD was positively correlated with 5-HT_{1A} binding potential in the PFC regions and in the raphe nuclei. These results suggest that lower levels of serotonin release at key brain projection sites such as the prefrontal regions may favor more severe suicidal ideation and higher-lethality suicide attempts.

5-HT_{2A} Receptors

5-HT_{2A} receptors have been the most studied serotonergic receptors in the brain of suicide victims. Using ^{3}H-spiperone as ligand, Stanley and Mann [18] reported that 5-HT_{2A} receptors are increased in Brodmann's areas 8 and 9 of suicide victims compared with normal control subjects. On the other hand, Owen et al. [19], who used ^{3}H-ketanserin as radioligand, did not find any significant differences in the PFC between suicide victims and normal control subjects. Subsequently, several studies examined 5-HT_{2A} receptors in postmortem brains of suicide victims and found them to be increased primarily in the PFC [20–23]. A few studies did not find any significant differences [24, 25]. On the other hand, one study found a decrease in ketanserin binding in the PFC of suicide victims [26] and two studies found a decrease in the hippocampus of suicide victims [24, 25]. Using ketanserin as ligand, more recently, Dean et al. [27] found that cortical HTR2A are lower in schizophrenia, MDD and people with mood disorders who died by suicide. It is difficult to assess the reasons for these differences in the 5-HT_{2A} receptor studies in the brains of suicide victims. Different ligands, specifically, spiperone, ketanserin and LSD, were used in these studies. Researchers who found an increase in 5-HT_{2A} receptors used spiperone and ketanserin, as well as LSD; therefore, these inconsistencies cannot be attributed to the difference in the ligands used for these studies. Differences in age, sex and axis I diagnosis may explain some of the discrepancies.

In addition to radioligand binding, we examined the protein and mRNA expression of 5-HT_{2A} receptors in Brodmann's area 9, the hippocampus and nucleus accumbens of teenage suicide victims [23]. We observed a significant increase in ^{125}I-LSD binding in the PFC of suicide victims. A significant increase in protein expression levels of 5-HT_{2A} receptors was noted in both the PFC and hippocampus of suicide victims; however, no such significant differences were found in the nucleus accumbens. Immunohistochemistry studies indicated that the expression of 5-HT_{2A} receptors was significantly greater in the pyramidal cells of layer V of the teenage suicide victims, whereas no changes were found in the pyramidal cells of other cortical layers (III and VI) or in the surrounding neuropil (layers IV, V, and VI). The increase in 5-HT_{2A} receptor protein was associated with increased mRNA expression in both the PFC and hippocampus. These changes were not associated with mental disorders. Using PET imaging, Soloff et al. [28] recently assessed the relationships between 5-HT_{2A} receptor function, gender and personality traits in borderline personality disorder, a disorder characterized by impulsive aggression and recurrent self-injurious or suicidal behavior. Region-specific differences were found in 5-HT_{2A} receptor binding related to diagnosis and gender, which predicted the clinical expression of aggression and impulsivity, suggesting that vulnerability to suicidal behavior in borderline personality disorder may be related to 5-HT_{2A} binding through the expression of personality risk factors.

5-HT_{2C} Receptors

Although the 5-HT_{2C} receptor has been shown to play a crucial role in regulating mood and anxiety, it has relatively been less studied in suicidal behavior. We were the first to examine 5-HT_{2C} receptors in postmortem brains of suicide subjects and reported that protein levels of 5-HT_{2C} receptors were higher in the PFC but not in the hippocampus or choroid plexus of suicide victims [29]. On the other hand, no significant differences in mRNA levels between suicide victims and control subjects were noted in these brain areas. Interestingly, transcripts of the gene encoding the 5-HT_{2C} receptor are modified by RNA editing, a posttranscriptional modification that converts adenosines to inosines. Compared with nonedited receptors, extensively edited receptor isoforms activate G protein less efficiently. Studies on mice revealed that 5-HT_{2C} pre-mRNA editing is regulated in a serotonin-dependent manner and postmortem studies on brain tissues of patients with schizophrenia and major depression found distinct site-specific alterations of 5-HT_{2C} editing in the PFC [30]. To date, the most complex alterations in 5-HT_{2C} pre-mRNA editing have been found in the brains of depressed suicide victims. In these brains, 5-HT_{2C} receptor isoforms with reduced functions are expressed at significantly increased levels, suggesting that the regulation of editing by synaptic serotonin is defective [31]. An examination of the efficiencies of RNA editing of the 5-HT_{2C} receptor in the PFC of control individuals versus subjects diagnosed with schizophrenia or MDD revealed no significant differences in RNA editing among the three populations. However, subjects who committed suicide exhibited a significant elevation of editing at the A site, which is predicted to change the amino acid sequence in the second intracellular loop of the 5-HT_{2C} receptor [32]. Gurevich et al. [33] found that in suicide victims who had a history of major depression, the pre-mRNA editing for the 5-HT_{2C} receptor at the C′ site was significantly increased, the editing at the D site was significantly decreased, and the C site showed a trend towards increased editing in the suicide victims compared with control subjects. Very recently, Di Narzo et al. [34] analyzed the connections among 5-HT_{2C} receptor editing, genome-wide gene expression and DNA methylation in suicide victims, individuals with MDD and nonpsychiatric controls. They found an overrepresentation of highly edited mRNA variants (which encode hypoactive 5-HT_{2C} receptors) in the brains of suicide victims. A large set of genes for which the expression level is associated with editing was detected. This signature set of editing-associated genes was significantly enriched for genes that are involved in synaptic transmission, genes that are preferentially expressed in neurons and genes whose expression is correlated with the level of DNA methylation. They also reported that the link between 5-HT_{2C} receptor editing and gene expression was disrupted in suicide victims. The results suggest that the postulated homeostatic function of 5-HT_{2C} receptor editing is dysregulated in individuals who committed suicide.

Noradrenergic System in Suicide

The role of the noradrenergic system in depression and suicide has been studied using blood, urine and CSF samples from depressed or suicidal patients, catecholamine depletion in living patients and postmortem brain tissues from depressed subjects and suicide victims. The major evidence implicating noradrenergic mechanisms in suicide is derived from the studies of a metabolite of norepinephrine known as 3-methoxy-4-hydroxyphenylglycol (MHPG) in the CSF of suicidal patients. It has been shown that low CSF MHPG predicts the risk of suicide attempts and the greater the MHPG deficiency the more lethal the suicide attempts [35]. On the other hand, the results from the studies of another metabolite, homovanillic acid, in CSF are mixed and only one of several studies demonstrated that low levels of CSF homovanillic acid were associated with suicidal behavior in patients with depressive illness [36]. Two studies reported that the 24-hour norepinephrine/epinephrine ratio in psychiatric patients with a history of suicide was lower than that of other psychiatric patients [37, 38]. Similarly, the studies of tyrosine hydroxylase in suicidal behavior showed inconsistent results. Whereas Arango et al. [39] found decreased numbers of locus coeruleus neurons, Ordway [40] found elevated tyrosine hydroxylase immunoreactivity and Biegon and Fieldust [41] reported decreased tyrosine hydroxylase immunoreactivity in these neuronal populations.

Adrenergic Receptors in Suicide

β-Adrenergic Receptors in Suicide

Noradrenergic receptors, particularly α_2- and β-adrenergic receptors, have received considerable attention in studies of postmortem brain pathology in suicide. One of the earliest studies determining the β-adrenergic receptor in postmortem brains of suicide victims was reported by Meyerson et al. [42]. Using ^{3}H-dihydroalprenolol (DHA, a β-adrenergic antagonist) as the ligand for β-adrenergic receptor binding, they did not find significant differences in the PFC of suicide victims, although there was a trend towards an increase in β-adrenergic receptor binding. On the other hand, Mann et al. [20] found a significant increase in DHA-specific binding in the frontal cortex of suicide victims, which was further supported by studies of Arango et al. [21] with similar findings. Autoradiographic studies also found a significant increase in β-adrenergic receptors in the gray matter outer layers and in the inner layers of the PFC and temporal cortex of suicide victims. Contrary to these reports, DePaermentier et al. [43] found decreased β-adrenergic receptors in the temporal cortex of suicide subjects. A similar finding was reported by Little et al. [44] using ^{125}I-pindolol as the radioligand. Thus, the results of studies of β-adrenergic receptors in postmortem brains of suicide victims appear to be mixed.

α-Adrenergic Receptors in Suicide

In contrast to β-adrenergic receptor, α-adrenergic receptors have been studied extensively in suicide brains. For example, using agonist binding for labeling α_2-adrenergic receptors, DePaermentier et al. [45] did not find any significant differences in the α_1- or α_{1D}- adrenergic receptors in the postmortem brains obtained from antidepressant-free suicide victims. Arango et al. [21] determined α_1-adrenergic receptors using prazosin as the radioligand and failed to find any difference in the PFC and temporal cortex of suicide victims. On the other hand, Gross-Isseroff et al. [46] found decreased α_1-adrenergic receptor binding in the PFC, temporal cortex and caudate nucleus of suicide victims. Gonzalez et al. [47] determined α_2-adrenergic receptors using the agonist ^{3}H-UK14304 in the hippocampus and frontal cortex and found a significant increase in the number of α_2-adrenergic receptors in the CA1 and dentate gyrus and in the external layers of the frontal cortex of suicide subjects. An increase in α_2-adrenergic receptors was also observed by Meana and Garcia-Sevilla [48] in the frontal cortex of suicide victims. Subsequent studies from this group showed increased protein and mRNA expression of α_2-adrenergic receptors in the PFC of suicide subjects. Ordway et al. [49] reported that only the agonist binding (^{125}I-iodoclonidine) to α_2-adrenergic receptors and not the antagonist binding (^{3}H-yohimbine) was greater in the locus coeruleus of suicide victims. Functional analyses suggest that α_2-adrenoceptor-linked $G_i\alpha$ signaling is increased in depressed suicide subjects [50], implicating this receptor in suicide. Underwood et al. [51] determined α_1- and α_2-adrenergic receptors using ^{3}H-prazosin and ^{3}H-p-aminoclonidine (^{3}H-PAC) by autoradiography in postmortem brains obtained from alcoholic suicide and alcoholic nonsuicide subjects, as well as normal control subjects. They found that the α_2-adrenergic receptors were decreased in alcoholic suicide victims in the dorsolateral frontal cortex and ventrolateral B46 and B47 of the PFC compared with control subjects. They also found that α_2-adrenergic receptors determined by autoradiography using ^{3}H-PAC were significantly decreased in B46/47 and B11 compared with control subjects.

Intracellular Signaling Mechanisms and Suicide

Downstream signal transduction pathways are important for behavioral and environmental adaptations by regulating neural plasticity and integrating various physiological processes, including modulation of neurotransmitter synthesis and release, regulation of receptors and ion channels, neuronal excitability, gene expression, and cell proliferation. Given the critical importance of intracellular signaling pathways, recent studies have focused on the role of various signaling molecules in the pathophysiology of suicide. The most studied intracellular signaling pathways in the pathophysiology of suicide are the PI and the adenylyl cyclase-cAMP pathways.

Phosphoinositide and Adenylyl Cyclase-cAMP Signaling Systems in Suicide
In the PI signaling pathway, agonist binding to neurotransmitter receptors such as 5-HT_{2A}, 5-HT_{2C} or α_1-adrenergic receptors causes activation of G proteins, which then activate the enzyme PI-specific phospholipase C (PI-PLC). PI-PLC then hydrolyzes phosphatidylinositol 4,5 biphosphate (PIP_2) and generates two intracellular second messengers – inositol 1,4,5 trisphosphate (IP_3) and diacylglycerol (DAG). DAG remains within the membrane and activates phospholipid- and calcium-dependent enzyme protein kinase C (PKC) and increases its affinity for calcium. PKC phosphorylates substrate proteins in the plasma membrane and cytosol. DAG is short lived and is rapidly phosphorylated to form phosphatidate by diacylglycerol kinase, thus causing the termination of PKC activation. The other second messenger, IP_3, leaves the cell membrane and diffuses within the cytosol. IP_3 then binds to IP_3 receptors and mobilizes Ca^{2+} from intracellular sources such as the endoplasmic reticulum. Once released, Ca^{2+} interacts with Ca^{2+}-sensitive calmodulin (CaM), which then activates calmodulin-dependent protein kinases (CaM kinases). PKC and CaM kinase can

activate transcription factors such as CREB. PKC has many substrates in cytosol where it can phosphorylate substrates, including MARCKS (fig. 1).

In the adenylyl cyclase-cAMP signaling system, agonist-induced modulation of G proteins causes the activation of adenylyl cyclase, which converts substrate ATP to cAMP. cAMP then activates phosphorylating enzyme protein kinase A (PKA). PKA, like PKC, activates several transcription factors, resulting in alterations in the transcription of genes. The intracellular level of cAMP is determined by the rate of its synthesis from ATP by adenylyl cyclase and its catabolic conversion to 5′ AMP by phosphodiesterases (fig. 1).

G Proteins in Suicide

Gα subunits have been classified into four major classes – G_s, G_i, G_q, and G_{12}. More than 16 distinct genes encode the G protein α subunits; 5 distinct β subunit genes and 12 γ subunit genes have also been identified [52]. $G_s\alpha$ stimulates adenylyl cyclase, whereas $G_i\alpha$ mediates the inhibition of adenylyl cyclase. $G_q\alpha$ is coupled to PLC, an enzyme that is involved in PI hydrolysis. $G_s\alpha$ and $G_i\alpha$ have also been shown to be operative in gating L-type Ca^{2+} channels and K^+ channels, respectively. A particular G protein can couple to more than one effector.

G protein function has been studied in the postmortem brains of suicide victims by several investigators. Cowburn et al. [53] found that basal and GTP-γ-S-stimulated adenylyl cyclase activity was significantly lower without any change in the expression of $G_s\alpha$ or $G_i\alpha$. The decreased GTP-γ-S-stimulated adenylyl cyclase activity was more profound in those suicide subjects who died from violence or had a history of depression. Pacheco et al. [54] found that GTP-γ-S-stimulated PI hydrolysis was decreased in the frontal cortex of depressed suicide subjects. In addition, they reported an increased expression of $G_s\alpha$ and a decreased expression of $G_{i2}\alpha$ in depressed suicide subjects. Gurguis et al. [55] found super-coupling of the receptors to the $G_s\alpha$ protein in the PFC of suicide subjects. Dowlatshahi et al. [56] did not find any significant differences in the protein expression of $G_s\alpha$ or $G_i\alpha$ in suicide subjects. Recently Valdizán et al. [50] reported that basal GTP-γ-S binding and cAMP accumulation did not differ but there were significant ^{35}S GTP-γ-S binding potency and maximal inhibition of AC activity in the suicide brain.

In a large postmortem brain study, we found that the levels of $G_{i2}\alpha$ and $G_o\alpha$ were decreased and the level of $G_s\alpha$-S was increased in the PFC of suicide subjects [57]. When suicide subjects were divided into subgroups of teenagers and adults, we observed that the mRNA levels of $G_{i2}\alpha$ and $G_o\alpha$ were significantly decreased and those of $G_s\alpha$-S were significantly increased in the PFC of adult suicide subjects, without any change in mRNA levels of $G_{i1}\alpha$. On the other hand, there were no significant differences in mRNA levels of any of the G protein subunits between teenage controls and teenage suicide subjects. Interestingly, in brains of depressed suicide subjects, we found that $G_s\alpha$ was less available for adenylyl cyclase signaling because of its presence in cytoskeletal-associated lipid raft-like domains, suggesting that membrane microdomains are critical in G protein signaling and are impaired in the suicide brain [58].

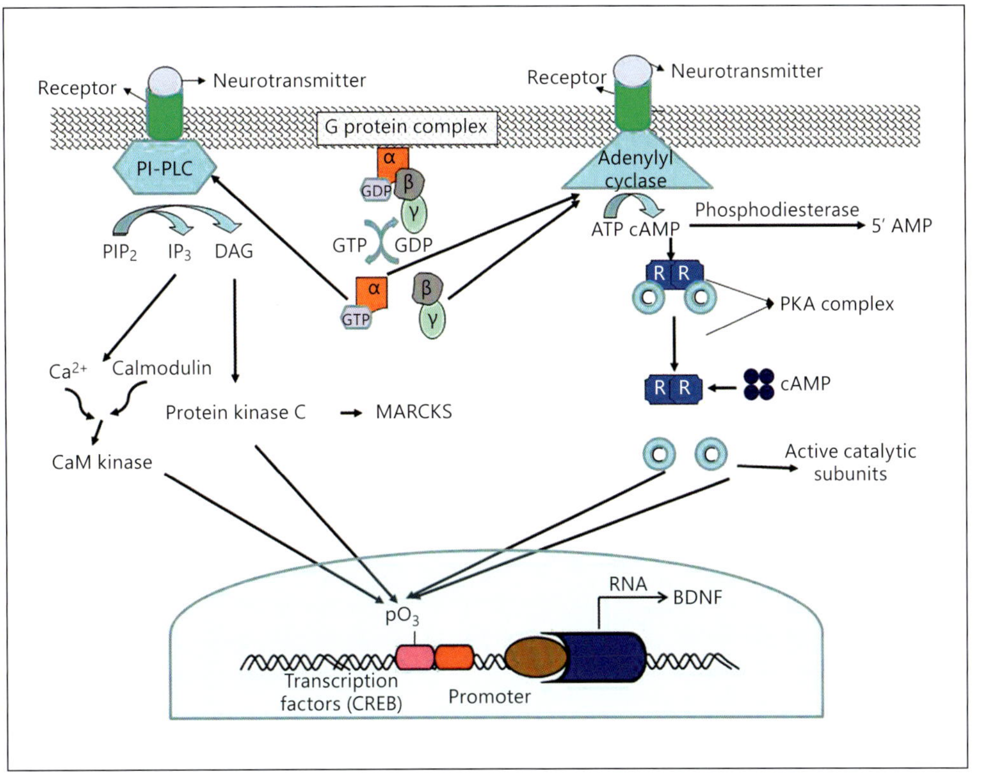

Fig. 1. Overview of G proteins, PI and adenylyl cyclase-cAMP signaling. R = Regulatory; C = catalytic. In the inactive state, the α subunit of G protein is bound to GDP and to βγ subunits. The binding of agonists to receptors causes an interaction of receptors with G proteins, which, in turn, releases GDP in exchange with GTP. This leads to the generation of α-GTP and a βγ subunit dimer. Both α and βγ subunits can interact with effectors. In the PI signaling pathway, the binding of neurotransmitter to G protein-coupled receptors leads to the activation of G proteins, which, in turn, activate enzyme PLC, which then converts PIP_2 into IP_3 and DAG. DAG then activates PKC and IP_3 binds to IP_3 receptors and mobilizes Ca^{2+} from intracellular sources such as the endoplasmic reticulum. Once released, Ca^{2+} interacts with CaM, which then activates CaM kinases. PKC and CaM kinases can then activate substrates such as CREB or MARCKS. In the adenylyl cyclase-cAMP signaling pathway, the binding of neurotransmitter to G protein-coupled receptors leads to the activation of G proteins, which, in turn, activate adenylyl cyclase, leading to the production of cAMP. PKA is a holoenzyme composed of two subunits: regulatory and catalytic. These regulatory and catalytic subunits form a tetrameric holoenzyme (R_2C_2). In the absence of cAMP, PKA exists as a stable inactive tetramer. The catalytic activity of cAMP is suppressed when the catalytic subunits form a complex with the regulatory subunits. c-AMP, generated in response to adenylyl cyclase activation, binds to the regulatory subunits of tetrameric PKA holoenzymes. The binding of cAMP to a regulatory subunit lowers its affinity for the catalytic subunit. This causes the release of free catalytic subunits. The catalytic subunit can catalyze phosphorylation of substrates in the cytoplasm or, after translocation of the catalytic subunits, in the nucleus. PKA is also anchored with A-kinase-anchoring proteins, causes compartmentalized localization of PKA and initiates phosphorylation of substrates in a localized fashion. As with PKC, PKA can activate CREB, which regulates the transcription of many neuronally expressed genes, including BDNF. Deactivation of PKA is achieved through the degradation of cAMP to 5′ AMP by cAMP-specific phosphodiesterases.

Phosphoinositide-Specific Phospholipase C and Protein Kinase C in Suicide

In the PI signaling, the enzyme PI-PLC converts PIP_2 into DAG and IP_3 and helps in the transduction of signals from the receptors to the nucleus (fig. 1). PI-PLC isoforms are classified into three major families – PLCβ, PLCγ and PLCδ. The PLCβ family consists of three members that are highly expressed in the brain – $PLCβ_1$, $PLCβ_2$ and $PLCβ_3$. PLCγ consists of $γ_1$ and $γ_2$ subunits, whereas PLCδ is subtyped into $δ_1$ and $δ_2$. Pacheco et al. [54] measured the expression levels of PLCβ in the PFC of depressed suicide victims but did not find any significant differences between suicide subjects and normal controls. In the PFC of teenage suicide, we observed that PI-PLC activity was significantly lower, which was associated with decreased expression of the $PLCβ_1$ isozyme [59].

PKC is the downstream regulatory enzyme in the PI pathway activated by DAG. The PKC family has been subgrouped into three classes – conventional (α, βI, βII, and γ), novel (δ, ε, η, and θ) and atypical (ι, κ, λ and τ). The conventional isozymes are phospholipid- and calcium-dependent, whereas the novel PKC isozymes do not require calcium for activation. The atypical isozymes are unresponsive to phorbol esters but can be activated by phosphatidylserine. We were the first to report that the binding of ^{3}H-PDBu to regulatory regions of PKC was decreased in the PFC of teenage suicide subjects, suggesting lower capability of PKA regulatory subunits to bind its activators [60]. In addition, we found that PKC activity was significantly decreased along with decreased expression of PKCα, βI, βII, and γ in both the PFC and hippocampus of teenage suicide subjects. In contrast, Coull et al. [61] did not find any change in ^{3}H-PBDu binding in antidepressant-treated suicide victims but noted increased ^{3}H-PBDu binding in antidepressant-free suicide victims. Using PCR and morphological microscopy observation, Lo Vasco et al. [62] recently examined the whole panel of expression of PLC isoforms in the brains of individuals who committed suicide and in normal controls in order to evaluate the involvement of specific PLC isoforms. They found that not only was the expression of PLC reduced but there was a complex disarrangement of the PLC panel of expression in suicide brains, with variable loss of expression of $PLCβ_1$, $PLCβ_3$, $PLCβ_4$, $PLCη_1$, and $PLCθ_1$. The most relevant differences were observed in the brains of the youngest (aged less than 29 years) suicide victims, which did not express a number of isoforms commonly detected in normal control brains. In this subgroup, from 2 to 4 out the commonly expressed 6 isoforms were not detected. These results suggest that the impaired expression of PLC enzymes worsens the signal transduction network in the brain, thus predisposing to suicidal behavior.

Myristoylated alanine-rich C kinase substrate (MARCKS), a major substrate of PKC, belongs to a family of homologous proteins that binds to calmodulin in a calcium-dependent manner. McNamara et al. [63] determined MARCKS expression in the PFC and hippocampus of suicide subjects and did not observe any differences. Similar to this study, we also did not find a change in the expression of MARCKS in the PFC of total suicide subjects [64]. However, we found that the expression of

MARCKS was increased in depressed suicide subjects but was decreased in nondepressed suicides. Interestingly, PKC-mediated phosphorylation of MARCKS was lower in the PFC of both depressed and nondepressed suicides. It appears that the PKC-mediated functional response at the level of MARCKS is abnormal in suicide subjects regardless of its expression level.

Protein Kinase A in Suicide

In the adenylyl cyclase-cAMP pathway, the effects of cAMP are primarily mediated by its receptor PKA. The activation of PKA is discussed in figure 1. In a comprehensive study, we examined PKA in the PFC of suicide victims [65, 66]. We observed that cAMP binding to regulatory subunits of PKA was decreased. However, there were no differences in the affinity of cAMP binding to these subunits. In addition, we observed that PKA activity was decreased in both the presence and the absence of cAMP, suggesting that decreased activation of PKA was not dependent on less availability of cAMP. This is a surprising finding given that $G_{i2}\alpha$ and $G_o\alpha$ were decreased and the level of $G_s\alpha$-S was increased in the brains of suicide subjects, suggesting greater availability of cAMP. Interestingly, we found that the expression of selective regulatory RIIβ and catalytic Cβ subunits was decreased in the PFC of suicide subjects, suggesting that decreases in cAMP binding and PKA activity could be due to decreases in the expression of these subunits. These results have been independently confirmed by Odagaki et al. [67].

In the teenage suicide population we found that PKA activity was decreased in the PFC. However, in contrast to the adult suicide population, teenage suicide subjects showed decreased expression of RIα and RIβ [60]. This is quite distinct from what we observed in the adult population. Why different regulatory and catalytic subunits are altered in teenage versus adult populations is not clear but could be related to specific behavioral characteristics such as affective disorders or impulsive aggressive behavior. Shelton et al. [68] reported that PKA activity is decreased in the PFC of depressed subjects. In another study, these investigators demonstrated that melancholic depressed subjects showed lower PKA RIα and Cβ expression in the frontal cortex, whereas those who died by suicide showed lower PKA RIα and Cα expression [69]. Thus, whether a decrease in specific PKA subunits is related to specific clinical phenotype needs to be further examined.

BDNF in Suicide

BDNF is a critical gene regulated by both PKA and PKC and participates in a wide range of physiological functions, including neurite outgrowth, phenotypic maturation, morphological plasticity, and synthesis of proteins for differentiated functioning of neurons and synapses. Our group was the first to examine the role of BDNF in suicide [70]. In this study, we found that the expression of BDNF was significantly lower in both the PFC and hippocampus of suicide subjects regardless of the psychiatric diagnosis. These results are further supported by a recent study which found decreased expression of BDNF in the hippocampus of suicide subjects [71]. Karege et al. [72] examined BDNF expression in 30 suicide victims and 24 drug-free nonsuicide subjects, who were devoid of psychiatric or neurological disease. They found a significant decrease in BDNF levels in the hippocampus and PFC, but not in the entorhinal cortex, of suicide victims who were drug free compared with nonsuicide controls. The decrease was observed in all suicide victims, regardless of diagnosis. This study supports a role of BDNF in the pathophysiological characteristics of suicidal behavior. It also suggests that a decrease in BDNF may be specific only to brain areas that are related to emotion and cognition. Karege et al. [72] also found that suicide subjects who were receiving antidepressant treatment did not show any change in the level of BDNF, suggesting that psychotropic drugs normalize the decreased level of BDNF in suicide subjects and that BDNF may be a mediator of psychotropic drug action. Interestingly, Kozicz et al. [73] examined the sex difference in the expression of BDNF in suicide subjects. They found that the BDNF level was much lower in the midbrain of male suicide subjects, whereas female suicide subjects showed an increased level of BDNF in this brain area, suggesting a possible sex effect in the regulation of BDNF expression in suicide subjects. Although the other studies did not find sex-specific changes in BDNF expression in the hippocampus or cortical areas of suicide subjects [70, 72], whether the sex-specific effect in BDNF expression is specific to the midbrain area needs to be further studied.

Because the epiphenomenon of teenage suicide may be different from that of adults, in a recent study we attempted to delineate the pathogenic mechanisms of adult versus teenage suicide [74]. We found that the expression of BDNF mRNA was decreased in the PFC and hippocampus of teenage suicide subjects. However, the protein expression of BDNF was decreased only in the PFC, not in the hippocampus. Thus, there is a disconnection between mRNA and protein expression of BDNF in the hippocampus of teenage suicide subjects. There is a possibility that differences in the expression of BDNF between the PFC and hippocampus of teenage suicide subjects could be associated with a defective translation or turnover of BDNF in the hippocampus.

Conclusion

In this chapter, we have critically discussed abnormalities associated with serotonergic and noradrenergic systems in suicide. It has been generally observed that suicidal behavior is associated with the presence of major mental disorders. Impulsive aggressive behavior and stress are also important risk factors for suicidal behavior. Since impulsive aggressive behavior, as well as stress, is implicated in abnormal serotonergic mechanisms, it is not surprising that the initial studies of neurobiological abnormalities in suicide focused on the serotonergic system. Overall, it appears that changes in serotonergic systems, particularly at the levels of 5-HT_{2A} and 5-HT_{1A} receptors, are quite consistent. The noradrenergic system, on the other hand, has not been studied as extensively as the serotonergic system and the findings are also mixed. However, at the downstream level, both these receptor systems show abnormalities in the brains of suicide subjects. The results indicate abnormalities in G proteins and of the effector molecule PLC as well as the phosphorylating enzymes PKA and PKC. The abnormalities in BDNF in suicide are compelling. Many postmortem brain studies consistently show decreased BDNF expression. One of the critical questions of these findings is whether the observed changes are specific to suicide, since the risk factors for suicide are not only the presence of major mental disorders – impulsive aggressive behavior and stress also play a critical role in suicidal behavior. The majority of the postmortem brain studies have been performed in samples obtained from depressed suicide subjects. Thus, it will be important to examine whether the observed changes are independent of depression or for that matter independent of psychiatric diagnosis.

Acknowledgments

The study was supported by grants to Dr. Yogesh Dwivedi from the National Institute of Mental Health (R01MH082802, R01MH100616, MH107183-01, and R01MH101980) and the American Foundation for Suicide Prevention.

References

1 Bach H, Huang YY, Underwood MD, Dwork AJ, Mann JJ, Arango V: Elevated serotonin and 5-HIAA in the brainstem and lower serotonin turnover in the prefrontal cortex of suicides. Synapse 2014;68:127–130.

2 Lesch KP, Wolozin BL, Murphy DL, Reiderer P: Primary structure of the human platelet serotonin uptake site: identity with the brain serotonin transporter. J Neurochem 1993;60:2319–2322.

3 Tuomisto J, Tukiainen E: Decreased uptake of 5-hydroxytryptamine in blood platelets from depressed patients. Nature 1976;262:596.

4 Meltzer HY, Arora RC, Baber R, Tricou BJ: Serotonin uptake in blood platelets of psychiatric patients. Arch Gen Psychiatry 1981;38:1322–1326.

5 Pandey GN, Dwivedi Y: Peripheral Biomarkers for Suicide; in Dwivedi Y (ed): The Neurobiological Basis of Suicide. Boca Raton, CRC Press, 2012.

6 Arango V, Underwood MD, Gubbi AV, Mann JJ: Localized alterations in pre- and postsynaptic serotonin binding sites in the ventrolateral prefrontal cortex of suicide victims. Brain Res 1995;688:121–133.

7 Arango V, Underwood MD, Mann JJ: Serotonin brain circuits involved in major depression and suicide. Prog Brain Res 2002;136:443–453.

8 Austin MC, O'Donnell SM: Regional distribution and cellular expression of tryptophan hydroxylase messenger RNA in postmortem human brainstem and pineal gland. J Neurochem 1999;72:2065–2073.

9 Arango V, Underwood MD, Boldrini M, Tamir H, Kassir SA, Hsiung S, Chen JJX, Mann JJ: Serotonin 1A receptors, serotonin transporter binding and serotonin transporter mRNA expression in the brainstem of depressed suicide victims. Neuropsychopharmacology 2001;25:892–903.

10 Okada S, Morinobu S, Fuchikami M, Segawa M, Yokomaku K, Kataoka T, Okamoto Y, Yamawaki S, Inoue T, Kusumi I, Koyama T, Tsuchiyama K, Terao T, Kokubo Y, Mimura M: The potential of SLC6A4 gene methylation analysis for the diagnosis and treatment of major depression. J Psychiatr Res 2014;53:47–53.

11 Middlemiss DN, Fozard JR. 8-hydroxy-2-(di-n-propylamino)-tetralin discriminates between subtypes of the 5-HT_1 recognition site. Eur J Pharmacol 1983;90:151–153.

12 Stockmeier CA, Shapiro LA, Dilley GE, Kolli TN, Friedman L, Rajkowska G: Increase in serotonin-1A autoreceptors in the midbrain of suicide victims with major depression-postmortem evidence for decreased serotonin activity. J Neurosci 1998;18:7394–7401.

13 Boldrini M, Underwood MD, Mann JJ, Arango V: Serotonin-1A autoreceptor binding in the dorsal raphe nucleus of depressed suicides. J Psychiatr Res 2008;42:433–442.

14 Joyce JN, Shane A, Lexow N, Winokur A, Casanova MF, Kleinman JE: Serotonin uptake sites and serotonin receptors are altered in the limbic system of schizophrenics. Neuropsychopharmacology 1993;8: 315–336.

15 Stockmeier CA, Dilley GE, Shapiro LA, Overholser JC, Thompson PA, Meltzer HY: Serotonin receptors in suicide victims with major depression. Neuropsychopharmacology 1997;16:162–173.

16 Dillon KA, Gross-Isseroff R, Israeli M, Biegon A: Autoradiographic analysis of serotonin 5-HT_{1A} receptor binding in the human brain postmortem: effects of age and alcohol. Brain Res 1991;554:56–64.

17 Sullivan GM, Oquendo MA, Milak M, Miller JM, Burke A, Ogden RT, Parsey RV, Mann JJ: Positron emission tomography quantification of $serotonin_{1A}$ receptor binding in suicide attempters with major depressive disorder. JAMA Psychiatry 2015;72:169–178.

18 Stanley M, Mann JJ: Increased serotonin-2 binding sites in frontal cortex of suicide victims. Lancet 1983; 1:214–216.

19 Owen F, Chambers DR, Cooper SJ, Crow TJ, Johnson JA, Lofthouse R, Poulter M: Serotonergic mechanisms in brains of suicide victims. Brain Res 1986; 362:185–188.

20 Mann JJ, Stanley M, McBride A, McEwen BS: Increased serotonin-2 and β-adrenergic receptor binding in the frontal cortices of suicide victims. Arch Gen Psychiatry 1986;43:954–959.

21 Arango V, Ernsberger P, Marzuk PM, Chen JS, Tierney H, Stanley M, Reis DJ, Mann JJ: Autoradiographic demonstration of increased serotonin 5-HT_2 and β-adrenergic receptor binding sites in the brain of suicide victims. Arch Gen Psychiatry 1990;47: 1038–1047.

22 Turecki G, Briere R, Dewar K, Antonetti T, Lesage AD, Seguin M, Chawky N, Vanier C, Alda M, Joober R, Benkelfat C, Rouleau GA: Prediction of level of serotonin 2A receptor binding by serotonin receptor 2A genetic variation in postmortem brain samples from subjects who did or did not commit suicide. Am J Psychiatry 1999;156:1456–1458.

23 Pandey GN, Dwivedi Y, Rizavi HS, Ren X, Pandey SC, Pesold C, Roberts RC, Conley RR: Higher expression of serotonin 5-HT_{2A} receptors in the postmortem brain of teenage suicide victims. Am J Psychiatry 2002;159:419–429.

24 Cheetham SC, Crompton MR, Katona CLE, Horton RW: Brain 5-HT_2 receptor binding sites in depressed suicide victims. Brain Res 1988;443:272–280.

25 Rosel P, Arranz B, San L, Vallejo J, Crespo JM, Uretavizcaya M, Navarro MA: Altered 5-HT_{2A} binding sites and second messenger inositol trisphosphate (PI_3) levels in hippocampus but not in frontal cortex from depressed suicide victims. Psychiatry Res 2000;99:173–181.

26 Gross-Isseroff R, Salama D, Israeli M, Biegon A: Autoradiographic analysis of [^{3}H]ketanserin binding in the human brain postmortem: effect of suicide. Brain Res 1990;507:208–215.

27 Dean B, Tawadros N, Seo MS, Jeon WJ, Everall I, Scarr E, Gibbons A: Lower cortical serotonin 2A receptors in major depressive disorder, suicide and in rats after administration of imipramine. Int J Neuropsychopharmacol 2014;17:895–906.

28 Soloff PH, Chiappetta L, Mason NS, Becker C, Price JC: Effects of serotonin-2A receptor binding and gender on personality traits and suicidal behavior in borderline personality disorder. Psychiatry Res 2014; 222:140–148.

29 Pandey GN, Dwivedi Y, Ren X, Rizavi HS, Faludi G, Sarosi A, Palkovits M: Regional distribution and relative abundance of $serotonin_{2c}$ receptors in human brain: effect of suicide. Neurochem Res 2006;3:167–176.

30 Sodhi MS, Burnet PW, Makoff AJ, Kerwin RW, Harrison PJ: RNA editing of the 5-HT_{2C} receptor is reduced in schizophrenia. Mol Psychiatry 2001;6:373–379.

31 Schmauss C: Regulation of serotonin 2C receptor pre-mRNA editing by serotonin. Int Rev Neurobiol 2005;63:83–100.

32 Niswender CM, Herrick-Davis K, Dilley GE, Meltzer HY, Overholser JC, Stockmeier CA, Emeson RB, Sanders-Bush E: RNA editing of the human serotonin 5-HT_{2C} receptor: alterations in suicide and implications for serotonergic pharmacotherapy. Neuropsychopharmacology 2001;24:478–491.

33 Gurevich I, Tamir H, Arango V, Dwork AJ, Mann JJ, Schmauss C: Altered editing of serotonin 2C receptor pre-mRNA in the prefrontal cortex of depressed suicide victims. Neuron 2002;34:349–356.

34 Di Narzo AF, Kozlenkov A, Roussos P, Hao K, Hurd Y, Lewis DA, Sibille E, Siever LJ, Koonin E, Dracheva S: A unique gene expression signature associated with serotonin 2C receptor RNA editing in the prefrontal cortex and altered in suicide. Hum Mol Genet 2014;23:4801–4813.

35 Lindqvist D, Janelidze S, Erhardt S, Träskman-Bendz L, Engström G, Brundin L: CSF biomarkers in suicide attempters – a principal component analysis. Acta Psychiatr Scand 2011;124:52–61.

36 Traskman-Bendz L, Asberg M, Bertilsson L, Thoren P: CSF monoamine metabolites of depressed patients during illness and after recovery. Acta Psychiatr Scand 1984;69:333–342.
37 Ostroff R, Giller E, Bonese K, Ebersole E, Harkness L, Mason J: Neuroendocrine risk factors of suicidal behavior. Am J Psychiatry 1982;139:1323–1325.
38 Prasad A: Neuroendocrine differences between violent and non-violent parasuicide. Abstracts Ann Meet Coll Int Neuropsychopharmacol, Florence, 1984, p 64.
39 Arango V, Underwood MD, Mann JJ: Fewer pigmented locus coeruleus neurons in suicide victims: preliminary results. Biol Psychiatry 1996;39:112–120.
40 Ordway GA: Pathophysiology of the locus coeruleus in suicide. Ann NY Acad Sci 1997;836:233–252.
41 Biegon A, Fieldust S: Reduced tyrosine hydroxylase immunoreactivity in locus coeruleus of suicide victims. Synapse 1992;10:79–82.
42 Meyerson LR, Wennogle LP, Abel MS, Cooper J, Lippa AS, Rauh CE, Beer B: Human brain receptor alterations in suicide victims. Pharmacol Biochem Behav 1982;17:159–163.
43 DePaermentier F, Cheetham SC, Crompton MR, Katona CLE, Horton RW: Brain β-adrenoceptor binding sites in antidepressant-free depressed suicide victims. Brain Res 1990;525:71–77.
44 Little KY, Clark TB, Ranc J, Duncan GE: β-adrenergic receptor binding in frontal cortex from suicide victims. Biol Psychiatry 1993;34:596–605.
45 DePaermentier F, Cheetham SC, Crompton MR, Katona CLE, Horton RW: Brain α_2-adrenoceptor binding sites in antidepressant-treated suicides and controls. Br J Pharmacol 1991;104:275P.
46 Gross-Isseroff R, Dillon KA, Fieldust SJ, Biegon A: Autoradiographic analysis of α_1-noradrenergic receptors in the human brain postmortem effect of suicide. Arch Gen Psychiatry 1990;47:1049–1053.
47 Gonzalez AM, Pascual J, Meana JJ, Barturen F, del Arco C, Pazos A, Garcia-Sevilla JA: Autoradiographic demonstration of increased α_2-adrenoceptor agonist binding sites in the hippocampus and frontal cortex of depressed suicide victims. J Neurochem 1994;63:256–265.
48 Meana JJ, Garcia-Sevilla JA: Increased α_2-adrenoceptor density in the frontal cortex of depressed suicide victims. J Neural Transm 1987;70:377–381.
49 Ordway GA, Widowson PS, Smith KS, Halaris A: Agonist binding to α_2-adrenoceptors is elevated in the locus coeruleus from victims of suicide. J Neurochem 1994;63:617–624.
50 Valdizán EM, Díez-Alarcia R, González-Maeso J, Pilar-Cuéllar F, García-Sevilla JA, Meana JJ, Pazos A: α_2-Adrenoceptor functionality in postmortem frontal cortex of depressed suicide victims. Biol Psychiatry 2010;68:869–872.
51 Underwood MD, Mann JJ, Arango V: Serotonergic and noradrenergic neurobiology of alcoholic suicide. Alcohol Clin Exp Res 2004;28(suppl 5):57S–69S.
52 Hildebrandt JD: Role of subunit diversity in signaling by heterotrimeric G proteins. Biochem Pharmacol 1997;54:325–339.
53 Cowburn RF, Marcusson JO, Eriksson A, Wiehager B, O'Neill C: Adenylyl cyclase activity and G-protein subunit levels in postmortem frontal cortex of suicide victims. Brain Res 1994;633;297–304.
54 Pacheco MA, Stockmeier C, Meltzer HY, Overholser JC, Dilley GE, Jope RS: Alterations in phosphoinositide signaling and G-protein levels in depressed suicide brain. Brain Res 1996;723:37–45.
55 Gurguis GN, Turkka J, Laruelle M, Kleinman J, Linnoila M: Coupling efficiency of brain β-adrenergic receptors to G_s protein in suicide, alcoholism and control subjects. Psychopharmacology (Berl) 1999;145:31–38.
56 Dowlatshahi D, MacQueen GM, Wang G, Reiach JS, Young LT: Protein-coupled cyclic AMP signaling in postmortem brain of subjects with mood disorders: effects of diagnosis, suicide, and treatment at the time of death. J Neurochem 1999;73:1121–1126.
57 Dwivedi Y, Rizavi HS, Conley RR, Roberts RC, Tamminga CA, Pandey GN: mRNA and protein expression of selective alpha subunits of G proteins are abnormal in prefrontal cortex of suicide victims. Neuropsychopharmacology 2002;27:499–517.
58 Donati RJ, Dwivedi Y, Roberts RC, Conley RR, Pandey GN, Rasenick MM: Postmortem brain tissue of depressed suicides reveals increased $G_s\alpha$ localization in lipid raft domains where it is less likely to activate adenylyl cyclase. J Neurosci 2008;28:3042–3050.
59 Pandey GN, Dwivedi Y, Pandey SC, Teas SS, Conley RR, Roberts RC, Tamminga CA: Low phosphoinositide-specific phospholipase C activity and expression of phospholipase C β_1 protein in the PFC of teenage suicide subjects. Am J Psychiatry 1999;156:1895–1901.
60 Pandey GN, Dwivedi Y, Ren X, Rizavi HS, Mondal AC, Shukla PK, Conley RR: Brain region specific alterations in the protein and mRNA levels of protein kinase A subunits in the post-mortem brain of teenage suicide victims. Neuropsychopharmacology 2005;30:1548–1556.
61 Coull MA, Lowther S, Katona CL, Horton RW: Altered brain protein kinase C in depression: a postmortem study. Eur Neuropsychopharmacol 2000;10:283–288.
62 Lo Vasco VR, Leopizzi M, Della Rocca C, Fais P, Montisci M, Cecchetto G: Impairment and reorganization of the phosphoinositide-specific phospholipase C enzymes in suicide brains. J Affect Disord 2015;174:324–328.

63 McNamara RK, Hyde TM, Kleinman JE, Lenox RH: Expression of the myristoylated alanine-rich C kinase substrate (MARCKS) and MARCKS-related protein (MRP) in the prefrontal cortex and hippocampus of suicide victims. J Clin Psychiatry 1999; 60(suppl 2):21–26.
64 Pandey GN, Dwivedi Y, Ren X, Rizavi HS, Roberts RC, Conley RR, Tamminga C: Altered expression and phosphorylation of myristoylated alanine-rich C kinase substrate (MARCKS) in postmortem brain of suicide victims with or without depression. J Psychiatr Res 2003;37:421–432.
65 Dwivedi Y, Conley RR, Roberts RC, Tamminga CA, Pandey GN: [^{3}H]cAMP binding sites and protein kinase A activity in the prefrontal cortex of suicide victims. Am J Psychiatry 2002;159:66–73.
66 Dwivedi Y, Rizavi HS, Shukla PK, Lyons J, Faludi G, Palkovits M, Sarosi A, Conley RR, Roberts RC, Tamminga CA, Pandey GN: Protein kinase A in postmortem brain of depressed suicide victims: altered expression of specific regulatory and catalytic subunits. Biol Psychiatry 2004;55:234–243.
67 Odagaki Y, García-Sevilla JA, Huguelet P, La Harpe R, Koyama T, Guimón J: Cyclic AMP-mediated signaling components are upregulated in the prefrontal cortex of depressed suicide victims. Brain Res 2001; 898:224–231.
68 Shelton RC, Sanders-Bush E, Manier DH, Lewis DA: Elevated 5-HT_{2A} receptors in postmortem prefrontal cortex in major depression is associated with reduced activity of protein kinase A. Neuroscience 2009;158:1406–1415.
69 Shelton RC, Hal, Manier D, Lewis DA: Protein kinases A and C in post-mortem prefrontal cortex from persons with major depression and normal controls. Int J Neuropsychopharmacol 2009;12: 1223–1232.
70 Dwivedi Y, Rizavi HS, Conley RR, Roberts, RC, Tamminga CA, Pandey GN: Altered gene expression of brain-derived neurotrophic factor and receptor tyrosine kinase B in postmortem brain of suicide subjects. Arch Gen Psychiatry 2003b;60:804–815.
71 Banerjee R, Ghosh AK, Ghosh B, Bhattacharyya S, Mondal AC: Decreased mRNA and protein expression of BDNF, NGF, and their receptors in the hippocampus from suicide: an analysis in human postmortem brain. Clin Med Insights Pathol 2013;6: 1–11.
72 Karege F, Vaudan G, Schwald M, Perroud N, La Harpe R: Neurotrophin levels in postmortem brains of suicide victims and the effects of antemortem diagnosis and psychotropic drugs. Brain Res Mol Brain Res 2005;136:29–37.
73 Kozicz T, Tilburg-Ouwens D, Faludi G, Palkovits M, Roubos E: Gender-related urocortin 1 and brain-derived neurotrophic factor expression in the adult human midbrain of suicide victims with depression. Neuroscience 2008;152:1015–1023.
74 Pandey GN, Ren X, Rizavi HS, Conley RR, Roberts RC, Dwivedi Y: Brain-derived neurotrophic factor and tyrosine kinase B receptor signalling in postmortem brain of teenage suicide victims. Int J Neuropsychopharmacol 2008;11:1047–1061.

Yogesh Dwivedi, PhD
Elesabeth Ridgely Shook Endowed Chair in Psychiatry, Professor of Psychiatry
Director of Translational Research, UAB Mood Disorder Program
Department of Psychiatry and Behavioral Neurobiology, University of Alabama at Birmingham
SC711 Sparks Center, 1720 2nd Avenue South
Birmingham, AL 35294–0017 (USA)
E-Mail ydwivedi@uab.edu

Kaschka WP, Rujescu D (eds): Biological Aspects of Suicidal Behavior.
Adv Biol Psychiatry. Basel, Karger, 2016, vol 30, pp 37–50 (DOI: 10.1159/000434736)

GABA, Depression and Suicide

Mohan Pabba[a] • Etienne Sibille[a–c]

[a]Neurobiology of Depression and Aging, Campbell Family Mental Health Research Institute, Centre for Addiction and Mental Health and Departments of [b]Psychiatry and [c]Pharmacology and Toxicology, University of Toronto, Toronto, Ont., Canada

Abstract

A significant proportion of patients diagnosed with major depressive disorder (MDD) encounter frequent hospitalization because of suicidal ideation or after attempting suicide. Moreover, a significant proportion of subjects with MDD commit suicide. As a result, MDD-related suicide is a leading cause of death globally and the main contributor to the number of deaths by suicide. However, the biological mechanisms underpinning both MDD-related and MDD-unrelated suicide remain elusive. Studies using human postmortem brain samples of MDD patients who died as a result of suicide suggest dysfunction of neurotransmitter systems, including the GABAergic systems at the biochemical, gene, cellular, brain area, and function levels. In this chapter, we review human postmortem studies on major depression from our research group, which suggest selective and robust alterations in the functioning of specific GABA-related genes. We then compare these findings between MDD subjects who died from suicide and those who died from other causes. Despite the low level of evidence provided by these studies in support of a dysfunction in the GABA system associated with suicide, we suggest that further and systematic molecular studies are needed to resolve the conflicting results reported in the literature. Moreover, clinical investigations using tools that directly engage cortical GABA function, such as transcranial magnetic stimulation, suggest that functional studies of the GABA system in clinical subjects may provide mechanistic insight and have potential therapeutic purpose.

Depression is a complex neuropsychiatric disorder. According to the *American Diagnostic and Statistical Manual of Mental Disorders*, 5th edition (DSM-5), depression is characterized by low mood or reduced interest towards pleasurable activities (anhedonia) and disturbances in cognitive (attention, concentration, recurrent suicidal thoughts) as well as somatic (weight, locomotor, sleep patterns) symptoms [1]. Based on the severity, recurrence and duration of episode characteristics, depression is further categorized into several distinct classes [1–3]. Epidemiological studies indicate that major depression or major depressive disorder (MDD) is the most prevalent among different classes of depression. It is estimated that about 17% of the US population and approximately 6.7% of the world's population (both men and women) are affected by MDD during their lifetime [3–5]. Interestingly, women experience MDD at a greater percentage than men. A significant proportion of patients diagnosed with MDD encounter frequent hospitalization because of suicidal ideation or after attempting suicide. Moreover, a significant proportion of subjects with MDD commit suicide [3, 6, 7]. As a result, MDD-related suicide is a leading cause of death globally and the main contributor to deaths by suicide [8]. However, the biological mechanisms underpinning both MDD-related and MDD-unrelated suicide remain elusive. Studies using human postmortem brain samples of MDD patients who died as a result of suicide suggest dysfunction of neurotransmitter systems, including the serotonergic and GABAergic systems at gene, cellular and network levels. Here we review human postmortem studies on major depression from our research group, which suggest selective and robust alterations in the functioning of specific GABA-related genes. We then compare these findings between MDD subjects who died from suicide and those who died from other causes. Aspects of this chapter have previously been presented elsewhere [9–11].

Brief Summary of Current Research on Suicide

Several models have been put forward in attempting to delineate the biological mechanisms underlying depression-mediated suicide [12, 13]. According to these models, suicide or suicidal attempt results from the interaction of distal and proximal risk factors [13]. The distal factors include familial and genetic predisposition, genetic variation and early-life adversity. These distal factors are of distant temporal time frame i.e. without any direct involvement, and predispose individuals to the development of suicidal behavior. On the other hand, proximal risk factors are often considered as the precipitating factors, which include alterations in the brain neurochemical compositions at a time point closer to the onset of the suicidal event [13]. Indeed, many postmortem examinations of brain tissue from depressed suicide victims suggest changes in several neurotransmitter systems, cellular signal transduction and neuroendocrine response [12–15]. The changes in neurotransmitter systems in the brain tissue of depressed suicide victims mostly include abnormalities in the serotonergic and GABAergic systems. The hypothesis that alterations in the serotonergic system are involved in suicide mainly came from the following seminal findings: (1) low cerebrospinal fluid levels of the serotonin metabolite 5-hydroxyindoleacetic acid (5-HIAA) [16] and (2) altered levels of serotonin receptor and uptake sites throughout the frontal cortex [17, 18] and in the midbrain serotonergic nuclei of suicide completers [19–22]. In spite of the vast literature suggesting the involvement of the serotonergic system in suicide, outstanding questions remain such as to what extent and how specific are those postmortem changes associated with suicidal behavior [13]. Several chapters of this book review the literature on genetics, epigenetics and cellular signal transduction pathways implicated in suicide.

Early Studies of the GABA System in Suicide

Multidisciplinary-based examinations performed on depressed suicide or control subjects have provided conflicting results for the involvement of GABAergic system components in depression-related suicide. For example, no differences were found in the levels of GABA either in the cerebrospinal fluid of individuals who attempted suicide or in the postmortem frontal cortex tissue of suicide victims who suffered from major or bipolar depression compared to subjects without a history of suicidality or normal controls [23, 24]. Similarly, neuropeptides expressed in GABA neurons, e.g. somatostatin (SST), neuropeptide Y (NPY) and GABA levels, were not significantly different between depressed patients who did or did not attempt suicide [25]. Interestingly, there were also no differences in neuropeptide levels in the cerebrospinal fluid of these patients in a 5-year follow-up study [25]. Sundman et al. [26] reported no differences between the depressed suicide victims and controls when GABA uptake sites were measured. In addition, no differences in the $GABA_B$ receptor levels were reported in the frontal cortex between depressed suicide and control subjects [27–29]. Similarly, an early study from our group also reported no differences in the expression of GABAergic components in the dorsolateral or orbital ventral prefrontal cortex, as tested by gene microarray analysis [30].

These results contrast with later reports suggesting alterations in the GABAergic system through targeted or large-scale investigations of gene expression profiles from postmortem brain tissue of individuals diagnosed with MDD and who died of suicide versus good mental health individuals who died of other causes [31, 32]. For instance, using qPCR-based analysis, the Anisman group observed a downregulation of $GABA_A$ receptor subunits mRNA levels in a region-dependent manner in depressed suicide victims [33, 34]. The same group also reported evidence suggesting increased methylation in the $GABA_A$ receptor promoter, as a potential molecular mechanism for the observed downregulated expression in suicide victims [35]. Two separate studies from the Turecki group revealed an altered expression of GABAergic components when analyzed for microarray-based global gene expression in suicide subjects with or without depression [31, 36]. By employing pathway analysis for microarray data, Zhurov et al. [37] suggested a wide range of perturbations in the gene expression that are required for synaptic activity, including GABAergic transmission in subjects diagnosed with MDD and who died of suicide. Another separate study reported that altered GABAergic transmission in suicide victims could result from alterations in the glutamate-GABA synthesis cycle [38].

Contrary to the above studies, by evaluating the changes in the levels of drug-binding sites e.g. benzodiazepine to $GABA_A$ receptors, Cheetham et al. [39] reported an increase in the $GABA_A$ receptors in the frontal cortex tissue of depressed suicide subjects. Choudary et al. [32] and Sequeira et al. [40], using gene microarray analysis, observed an upregulation of $GABA_A$ receptor subunits, specifically

$GABA_A$ α1 and $GABA_A$ β3 in specific cerebral cortical areas of subjects with depressive symptoms and who committed suicide. Lee et al. [41] found an increase in the cerebrospinal fluid GABA levels with personality-disordered subjects who had a history of suicidal behavior. The summary of these findings suggests a complex picture and it is not clear whether the inconsistent results reflect the inherent variability across depressed populations or the lack of common molecular techniques to assess the underlying neurobiology.

GABA in Depression: Evidence from Human Postmortem Studies from Our Research Group

Molecular and cellular evidence from postmortem studies and in combination with in vivo imaging data suggests alterations in several components of the local cell circuitry in MDD [9, 10]. These components include deregulated GABA and glutamate homeostasis, specifically changes to the structure and function of glutamatergic neurons, dendritic-targeting GABAergic neurons, astrocytes, and oligodendrocytes. Based on our findings which we have summarized elsewhere [10], a hypothetical set of events contributing to disrupted processing and altered transfer of synaptic information in depression may occur in corticolimbic circuits, as follows: (1) changes in pyramidal neuron structure and in the availability of glutamate could disrupt the synaptic transfer of information; (2) reduced inhibition by dendritic targeting SST-positive GABA interneurons may lead to suboptimal modulation of excitatory postsynaptic signals onto dendritic spines; (3) suboptimal conduction of action potentials along the pyramidal axon could be caused by decreased oligodendrocyte support, leading to decreased integrity of information input or output, and (4) impaired astrocyte function may cause altered extracellular neurotransmitter clearance and recycling, which in turn may lead to an imbalance in GABA and glutamate homeostasis within their respective tripartite synapses [10]. Evidence from studies performed on corticolimbic regions of human postmortem brains by our group suggests a robust effect of depression on the GABA component, specifically affecting dendritic inhibition.

Reduced Markers of GABA-Related Dendritic Inhibition in Major Depression

GABA-positive neurons can be divided into subgroups based on morphology, neuropeptides that they express, electrophysiological properties, and the cellular compartments they target. GABA neurons expressing SST, NPY and cortistatin (CORT) target and inhibit the dendrites of pyramidal neurons, whereas interneurons expressing parvalbumin and cholecystokinin target the cell body and axon initial segment. Vasoactive intestinal peptide or calretinin-expressing neurons inhibit other

GABA neurons. Reduced density of GABA neuronal immunoreactivity for specific calcium-binding proteins has been reported in the dorsolateral prefrontal cortex (dlPFC) in major depression [42]; however, for contrary findings, see also [43, 44]. The density of calbindin-positive neurons was reduced by 50% in the dlPFC and no differences in parvalbumin-positive neurons were observed. Reductions in the density of calbindin-positive neurons were also reported in the occipital cortex [45].

We have reported a reduction in the expression of SST in the dlPFC [46], subgenual anterior cingulate cortex (sgACC) [47, 48] and amygdala [49] of subjects with MDD. These findings are consistent with previous studies, as SST is mostly expressed in calbindin-positive cells in the cortex [50]. NPY and CORT expression was also lower in the sgACC and amygdala in subjects with major depression [48, 49]. In contrast, cholecystokinin and calretinin were unaffected in the ACC and amygdala, while parvalbumin expression was lower in the ACC but not in the dlPFC [46, 48]. Altogether, these results suggest a common effect on markers of GABA neurons specifically inhibiting the dendrites of excitatory pyramidal neurons.

On the other hand, reduced gene expression levels of GAD67, an enzyme responsible for the synthesis of GABA from glutamate, have not been consistently reported but were observed in some studies, including at the protein level in the dlPFC [51] and at the mRNA levels coding for both GAD65 and GAD67 in the sgACC [48]. These cellular findings are consistent with reports of decreased GABA concentration in major depression, as observed by ^{1}H-MRS (proton magnetic resonance spectroscopy) or by transcranial magnetic stimulation (TMS) of the occipital and frontal cortices [52–55]. Selective serotonin reuptake inhibitors or electroconvulsive therapy reverse these changes [56, 57]. The combined functional imaging and resting-state MRS studies have suggested that the concentration of GABA in the ACC mediates the responses of the default mode network during emotion processing [58] and, intriguingly, reduced GABA levels in the ACC correlate with measures of anhedonia across depressed and control adolescents [54]. These brain-based observations in human subjects with MDD provide evidence for the GABA hypothesis of emotion dysregulation in depression [59, 60] which was originally proposed in 1980 based on the efficacy of sodium valproate, a GABAergic anticonvulsant, in the treatment of mania [61]. This was further supported by various reports demonstrating low GABA levels in the plasma and cerebrospinal fluid of subjects with psychiatric illnesses, including major depression [62–65], and later by the association between GABAergic transmission and control of stress [for review, see 60], by the effect of monoaminergic antidepressants on GABAergic transmission [56], and genetic manipulation studies in rodents [66]. Taken together, these studies provide compelling evidence for reduced GABA levels and selective cellular changes that potentially affect neuropeptide-related and/or GABA-related functions, specifically those involving the regulation of information input onto pyramidal neurons (dendritic tree).

A Model Linking Reduced GABA-Mediated Dendritic Inhibition with Increased Focus on the Self in Major Depression

Taking into account the available literature on altered GABA function in depression, we recently proposed a working model that links our molecular and cellular findings from human postmortem brain tissue with brain imaging findings, psychological concepts and all the way to symptom dimension [9]. Specifically, selective changes in the GABA-related inhibitory components of the input/output regulation of excitatory pyramidal cell function, combined with anatomical and connectivity differences between the ACC and dlPFC, may underlie the observed opposite functional changes between those two regions in MDD and the associated shift in neural network activities that include those regions (increased default mode and decreased executive network function). The resultant changes in integrated brain function may then emerge as a critical shift in awareness, specifically in the balance from external to internal mental focus. This is reflected by unspecific somatic symptoms and the predominance of the own cognitions manifested in increased self-focus, hence potentially underlying the common symptom of rumination that plagues many MDD patients [for further details, see 9]. Therefore, restoring GABA-mediated dendritic inhibitory function may reduce pyramidal cell activation and the excitatory tone, contributing to reduced ACC activation with a positive response to therapeutic intervention such as deep brain stimulation, for instance [67].

It is interesting to note that cortical inhibitory deficits are frequent across neuropsychiatric disorders. For instance, alterations in SST levels have also been identified in schizophrenia [68], bipolar disorder [69, 70], Huntington's disease [71], Alzheimer's disease [72, 73], and Parkinson's diseases [74]. This could suggest the presence of intrinsic vulnerability factors within SST and related GABA neurons and that common biological insults may similarly affect this cell population across several brain disorders [75]. Accordingly, using genetic and environmental stress models in mice, we recently identified the basic cellular mechanism of endoplasmic reticulum-mediated unfolded protein response as a putative cellular mechanism underlying the vulnerability of SST neurons to physiological and psychosocial stress [76]. It is not known whether this mechanism occurs in human SST neurons but one can speculate that those intrinsic cellular vulnerabilities may represent a common biological mechanism for deficits in SST-mediated GABA function across disorders and may in fact underlie the mood component (depressive symptoms) across neuropsychiatric disorders. We discuss this hypothesis in more details in the study by Lin and Sibille [75]. Moreover, with regard to suicidality and based on the GABA, self-awareness and depression model described earlier in this chapter, those common cellular and molecular deficits could also be linked to the negative cognitive processes associated with increased self-awareness and self-focus that may contribute to suicidal tendencies across neuropsychiatric disorders. We next review our past studies and the broader literature in search for evidence in support of this premise.

Somatostatin-Related GABA Measures in Major Depressive Disorder According to Suicide Status

In the literature, death by suicide has been previously associated with reduced BDNF expression [77–79] (see also chapter by Richard-Devantoy and Courtet, this vol., pp. 88–100). Suicide victims exhibit low hippocampal and midbrain BDNF levels [79], reduced activity-dependent BDNF expression, possibly through hypermethylation of BDNF promoter/exon IV [80], and increased risk for violent suicide in BDNF Met allele carriers [81, 82]. Do the cellular and molecular changes we reported in MDD, as described in the previous sections of this chapter, support a role for those changes in suicide when reanalyzed according to suicide status? Two of our studies provide enough data to investigate this question.

In the first study we tested the hypothesis that the illness may be associated with robust molecular changes in depressed suicide subjects and we investigated large-scale gene expression in the postmortem brains of 21 MDD female subjects paired with matched controls [49]. We focused on the lateral, basolateral and basomedial complex of nuclei of the amygdala as a neural hub of mood regulation affected in MDD. The most robust finding that we observed was the downregulation of gene transcripts encoding for GABA interneuron-related peptides, including SST, NPY and CORT, in a pattern reminiscent of that previously reported in mice with low BDNF [83, 84]. BDNF itself was significantly downregulated at the RNA and protein levels in MDD subjects. This pattern of gene expression changes was recapitulated in mice with a constitutive (BDNF heterozygous) or activity-dependent (exon IV knockout) decrease in BDNF function, with a common effect on SST and NPY. Collectively, the above observations provide direct (low RNA/protein) and indirect (low BDNF-dependent gene pattern) evidence for reduced BDNF function in the amygdala of female subjects with MDD [49]. The observation of reduced BDNF function is specifically interesting with respect to our hypothesis linking reduced BDNF to suicidality, since altered BDNF structure and function have been reported in depressed suicide victims [77–79, 85]. When splitting the sample according to death by suicide or other means, we observed that BDNF mRNA and pro-BDNF protein levels were further, although nonsignificantly, decreased in depressed suicide victims [mRNA: $\log_2$ (suicide/controls ratio) = –0.41 vs. –0.28 for nonsuicide MDD patients compared to matched controls, $p = 0.34$; pro-BDNF protein: $\log_2$ (suicide/controls ratio) = –0.62 vs. –0.47 for nonsuicide MDD patients compared to matched controls, $p = 0.28$]. However, we also observed reduced effect sizes on BDNF-dependent and GABA-related genes in suicide versus nonsuicide MDD subjects (fig. 1). Note that these results were not significant, potentially due to reduced sample size. Nevertheless, the observed direction of effects in the depressed suicide group does not provide sufficient evidence in support of a greater effect of GABA dysfunction associated with suicide status.

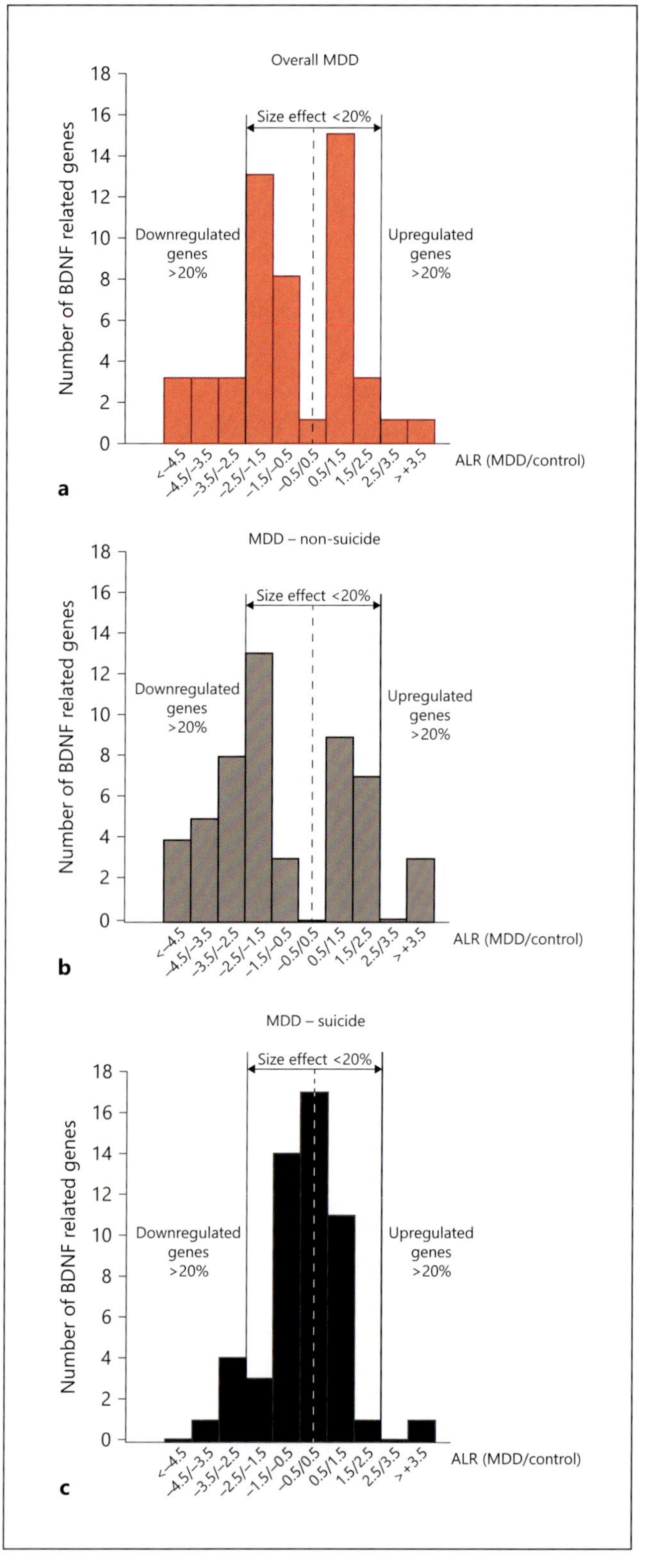

Fig. 1. GABA-related gene expression changes in the amygdala of depressed subjects who died by suicide compared to subjects who died from other causes. ALR = Average log ratio. Distribution histograms of 52 BDNF-related genes, including many GABA-related genes, depending on their changes in the overall MDD population (**a**), in MDD subjects who died by accidental or natural causes (n = 14; **b**) and MDD subjects who died by suicide (n = 7; **c**). The values are in $\log_2$ of the corresponding group ratios. The narrowing of the histogram around the no-change axis indicates a higher frequency of BDNF-dependent and GABA-related genes with low values in suicide MDD subjects (n = 7) compared to the nonsuicide MDD subjects (**b**). The figure has been reproduced with permission from Guilloux et al. [49].

Table 1. Suicide effect on BDNF and BDNF-dependent GABA-related gene expression in the sgACC of depressed subjects who died by suicide compared to subjects who died from other causes

	All		MDD and suicide		MDD not suicide	
	ALR	p value	ALR	p value	ALR	p value
TrkB	–0.52	0.003[a]	–0.51	0.039	–0.52	0.015[a]
CORT	–0.58	1.69E–05[a]	–0.54	0.002[a]	–0.68	2.63E–06[a]
VGF	–0.63	0.001[a]	–0.69	0.007	–0.58	0.010[a]
SST	–0.59	0.001[a]	–0.04	0.861	–0.83	0.005[a]
TAC1	–0.42	0.016	–0.26	0.285	–0.55	0.008[a]
NPY	–0.66	1.01E–04[a]	–0.53	0.015	–0.72	4.25E–05[a]
SNAP25	–0.69	4.53E–04[a]	–0.82	0.008	–0.65	0.001[a]
GAD2 (GAD65)	–0.48	2.00E–03[a]	–0.37	0.116	–0.54	0.001[a]
GAD1 (GAD67)	–0.41	1.00E–03[a]	–0.43	0.019	–0.40	0.003[a]
PVALB (PV)	–0.58	0.005[a]	–0.86	0.004[a]	–0.42	0.038[a]

Changes in suicide and nonsuicide MDD subjects for genes with significant MDD effects are shown. ALR = Average log ratio. $p < 0.05$: statistically significant. The table has been reproduced with permission from Tripp et al. [48].
[a] Significance after correction for multiple testing.

In the second study, we used quantitative PCR to assess the gene expression of BDNF and the same GABA-related genes in the sgACC in a large cohort of postmortem MDD and control subjects (n = 51/group; 49% female) [48]. Parallel studies in mice with reduced BDNF function confirmed the BDNF dependency on many of the relevant GABA markers in this brain region. In MDD, BDNF itself was unchanged but the expression of its main receptor (TrkB, tropomyosin-related kinase B) was reduced. Genes with demonstrated BDNF dependency, including markers of dendritic-targeting interneurons (SST, NPY, CORT) and a GABA synthesizing enzyme (GAD2), were robustly downregulated in the combined MDD cohort, together suggesting reduced neurotrophic function in MDD affecting multiple aspects of the GABA inhibitory local cell circuit. However, when splitting the sample by suicide status in this study, the observed gene expression differences appeared less robust in MDD subjects who died by suicide compared to MDD subjects who died by other causes (table 1). Therefore, similar to the first study performed in the amygdala, results in the ACC of depressed suicide group do not provide sufficient evidence to support a greater effect of GABA dysfunction associated with suicide status. However, do the above-described molecular studies preclude any role for GABA in suicidality? We believe that additional studies need to be performed on multiple molecular and cellular components of the GABA system in suicidal victims in the context of other psychiatric disorders, since taken together the literature is currently inconclusive on this topic.

GABA, Transcranial Magnetic Stimulation and Suicide

What other source of information provide putative links between altered GABA function and suicidality? Interestingly, recent studies using neurostimulation techniques such as TMS are emerging as therapeutic approaches not only as antidepressant but also to potentially protect subjects against suicidal ideation, suicide attempts and eventually suicide deaths. TMS is a safe and noninvasive method that delivers small focal varying frequencies of currents to the brain regions (e.g. dlPFC in the case of depressed subjects) under the dynamic magnetic field [86–88]. Several studies have shown TMS as an effective treatment therapy for reducing apathy and decreasing suicidal ideations. For example, repeated TMS treatment for multiple days in several sessions was found to be safe and decreased suicidal ideations in depressed suicide subjects [89, 90]. Repetitive prefrontal TMS on patients suffering from treatment-resistant MDD and having prior suicidal ideation experienced reduced suicidal thinking after the treatment [91]. A separate prefrontal repetitive TMS study recently concluded by George et al. [92] on 41 subjects who had been admitted to hospital based on suicidal thoughts out of a large pool of enrolled inpatients showed a rapid antisuicide effect after the treatment, although the TMS effect did not differ from sham treatment over the 3 days of the treatment. Notably, in contrast to antidepressant medications such as selective serotonin reuptake inhibitors, none of these TMS studies reported increases in suicidal thoughts. Though there are several studies demonstrating the efficacy of TMS in treating patients with suicidal thoughts, it is important to note that TMS is not directly intervening in suicidal ideation or behavior [88]. Rather, TMS might actually modulate the preconditions that are associated with suicidality, e.g. depression [93, 94].

How do these TMS studies relate to putative GABA function in depression and in suicidality? Although the mechanisms by which TMS exerts antidepressant effects and potentially reduce suicidality remain obscure, TMS represents a noninvasive technique to measure cortical inhibition and associated GABA function. TMS has been used to measure neurophysiological features of brain functions such as short-interval cortical inhibition and cortical silent period [95, 96]. Pharmacological manipulations suggest that these measure GABAergic inhibitory neurotransmission related to $GABA_A$ and $GABA_B$ receptor-mediated neurotransmission [97–99]. Reduced cortical inhibition has been reported by TMS in depression [53]. Moreover, since TMS signal is thought to only penetrate the superficial cortical layers, we could speculate that it may selectively affect the GABAergic fibers that populate those superficial layers, namely fibers from the traditional Martinotti cells, which represent a main subgroup of SST-positive neurons – the same neurons we discussed earlier in this chapter. Thus, one could speculate that TMS may exert antidepressant activity through the modulation and recruitment of GABA neurons that are otherwise affected in depression, as measured in the postmortem brain. Indeed, preliminary studies showing a role for TMS in reducing suicidality [91, 92] suggest that this effect may be similarly mediated by boosting GABA function [100, 101].

Conclusion

As discussed in this chapter, reduced GABA function in depression can be linked from the molecular and cellular levels all the way to the symptom of exaggerated self-focus and potential rumination in depression [9]. However, those molecular and cellular changes appear less robust in samples from depressed subjects who died by suicide. Moreover, without control groups of subjects who committed suicide in the absence of depression, one cannot conclude that these findings reflect a pathology (or lack of it) associated with suicide itself rather than a subtype of depression characterized by death by suicide. Nonetheless, despite the low level of evidence provided by these studies in support of a dysfunction in the GABA system associated with suicide, we suggest that further molecular studies are needed to resolve the conflicting results reported in the literature. Results from studies using TMS in depression suggest a potential role in reducing suicidal thoughts and suicidality. Therefore, since TMS directly engages cortical GABA function, further functional studies of the GABA system in live patients, using TMS, may provide mechanistic insight and have potential therapeutic purpose.

Acknowledgments

This work was supported by National Institute of Mental Health grant R01MH077159 (E.S.). The funding agencies had no role in the study design, data collection and analysis, decision to publish, or preparation of the manuscript. The authors declare no conflicts of interest. We thank Mehrab Ali for careful feedback on the manuscript.

References

1 American Psychiatric Association: The Diagnostic and Statistical Manual of Mental Disorders: DSM-V-TR, ed 5. Washington, APA, 2013.
2 WHO: International Classification of Mental and Behavioral Disorders, ed 10, rev. Geneva, WHO, 1992.
3 Friedman ES: Handbook of Depression, ed 2. London, Springer, 2014, pp 1–11.
4 Kessler RC, et al: Lifetime prevalence and age-of-onset distributions of DSM-IV disorders in the National Comorbidity Survey Replication. Arch Gen Psychiatry 2005;62:593–602.
5 Waraich P, et al: Prevalence and incidence studies of mood disorders: a systematic review of the literature. Can J Psychiatry 2004;49:124–138.
6 Bostwick JM, Pankratz VS: Affective disorders and suicide risk: a reexamination. Am J Psychiatry 2000; 157:1925–1932.
7 Harris EC, Barraclough B: Suicide as an outcome for mental disorders. A meta-analysis. Br J Psychiatry 1997;170:205–228.
8 WHO: The Global Burden of Disease – 2004 update. Geneva, WHO, 2004.
9 Northoff G, Sibille E: Why are cortical GABA neurons relevant to internal focus in depression? A cross-level model linking cellular, biochemical and neural network findings. Mol Psychiatry 2014;19: 966–977.
10 Beverly French, Seney ML, Sibille E: Altered GABA function in major depression; in Popoli M, Diamond D, Sanacora G (eds): Synaptic Stress and Pathogenesis of Neuropsychiatric Disorders. New York, Springer, 2014, pp 203–223.
11 Sibille E, French B: Biological substrates underpinning diagnosis of major depression. Int J Neuropsychopharmacol 2013;16:1893–1909.

12 Mann JJ: Neurobiology of suicidal behaviour. Nat Rev Neurosci 2003;4:819–828.
13 Turecki G: The molecular bases of the suicidal brain. Nat Rev Neurosci 2014;15:802–816.
14 Pandey GN, et al: Protein kinase C in the postmortem brain of teenage suicide victims. Neurosci Lett 1997;228:111–114.
15 Roy A: Hypothalamic-pituitary-adrenal axis function and suicidal behavior in depression. Biol Psychiatry 1992;32:812–816.
16 Asberg M, et al: 'Serotonin depression' – a biochemical subgroup within the affective disorders? Science 1976;191:478–480.
17 Stanley M, Virgilio J, Gershon S: Tritiated imipramine binding sites are decreased in the frontal cortex of suicides. Science 1982;216:1337–1339.
18 Stanley M, Mann JJ: Increased serotonin-2 binding sites in frontal cortex of suicide victims. Lancet 1983; 1:214–216.
19 Underwood MD, et al: Neuron density and serotonin receptor binding in prefrontal cortex in suicide. Int J Neuropsychopharmacol 2012;15:435–447.
20 Parsey RV, et al: Lower serotonin transporter binding potential in the human brain during major depressive episodes. Am J Psychiatry 2006;163:52–58.
21 Arango V, Underwood MD, Mann JJ: Serotonin brain circuits involved in major depression and suicide. Prog Brain Res 2002;136:443–453.
22 Mann JJ, Brent DA, Arango V: The neurobiology and genetics of suicide and attempted suicide: a focus on the serotonergic system. Neuropsychopharmacology 2001;24:467–477.
23 Korpi ER, Kleinman JE, Wyatt RJ: GABA concentrations in forebrain areas of suicide victims. Biol Psychiatry 1988;23:109–114.
24 Berrettini WH, et al: Cerebrospinal fluid studies of bipolar patients with and without a history of suicide attempts. Ann NY Acad Sci 1986;487:197–201.
25 Roy A: Neuropeptides in relation to suicidal behavior in depression. Neuropsychobiology 1993;28: 184–186.
26 Sundman I, et al: GABA uptake sites in frontal cortex from suicide victims and in aging. Neuropsychobiology 1997;35:11–15.
27 Cross JA, et al: Brain $GABA_B$ binding sites in depressed suicide victims. Psychiatry Res 1988;26:119–129.
28 Arranz B, et al: Gamma-aminobutyric acid-B ($GABA_B$) binding sites in postmortem suicide brains. Neuropsychobiology 1992;26:33–36.
29 Gonzalez-Maeso J, et al: Neurotransmitter receptor-mediated activation of G-proteins in brains of suicide victims with mood disorders: selective supersensitivity of α_{2A}-adrenoceptors. Mol Psychiatry 2002;7:755–767.
30 Sibille E, et al: Gene expression profiling of depression and suicide in human prefrontal cortex. Neuropsychopharmacology 2004;29:351–361.
31 Sequeira A, et al: Global brain gene expression analysis links glutamatergic and GABAergic alterations to suicide and major depression. PLoS One 2009;4: e6585.
32 Choudary PV, et al: Altered cortical glutamatergic and GABAergic signal transmission with glial involvement in depression. Proc Natl Acad Sci U S A 2005;102:15653–15658.
33 Merali Z, et al: Dysregulation in the suicide brain: mRNA expression of corticotropin-releasing hormone receptors and $GABA_A$ receptor subunits in frontal cortical brain region. J Neurosci 2004;24: 1478–1485.
34 Poulter MO, et al: Altered organization of $GABA_A$ receptor mRNA expression in the depressed suicide brain. Front Mol Neurosci 2010;3:3.
35 Poulter MO, et al: $GABA_A$ receptor promoter hypermethylation in suicide brain: implications for the involvement of epigenetic processes. Biol Psychiatry 2008;64:645–652.
36 Klempan TA, et al: Altered expression of genes involved in ATP biosynthesis and GABAergic neurotransmission in the ventral prefrontal cortex of suicides with and without major depression. Mol Psychiatry 2009;14:175–189.
37 Zhurov V, et al: Molecular pathway reconstruction and analysis of disturbed gene expression in depressed individuals who died by suicide. PLoS One 2012;7:e47581.
38 Bernstein HG, et al: Disruption of glutamate-glutamine-GABA cycle significantly impacts on suicidal behaviour: survey of the literature and own findings on glutamine synthetase. CNS Neurol Disord Drug Targets 2013;12:900–913.
39 Cheetham SC, et al: Brain GABAA/benzodiazepine binding sites and glutamic acid decarboxylase activity in depressed suicide victims. Brain Res 1988;460: 114–123.
40 Sequeira A, et al: Patterns of gene expression in the limbic system of suicides with and without major depression. Mol Psychiatry 2007;12:640–655.
41 Lee R, Petty F, Coccaro EF: Cerebrospinal fluid GABA concentration: relationship with impulsivity and history of suicidal behavior, but not aggression, in human subjects. J Psychiatr Res 2009;43:353–359.
42 Rajkowska G, et al: GABAergic neurons immunoreactive for calcium binding proteins are reduced in the prefrontal cortex in major depression. Neuropsychopharmacology 2007;32:471–482.
43 Beasley CL, et al: Selective deficits in prefrontal cortical GABAergic neurons in schizophrenia defined by the presence of calcium-binding proteins. Biol Psychiatry 2002;52:708–715.

44 Cotter D, et al: The density and spatial distribution of GABAergic neurons, labelled using calcium binding proteins, in the anterior cingulate cortex in major depressive disorder, bipolar disorder, and schizophrenia. Biol Psychiatry 2002;51:377–386.
45 Maciag D, et al: Reduced density of calbindin immunoreactive GABAergic neurons in the occipital cortex in major depression: relevance to neuroimaging studies. Biol Psychiatry 2010;67:465–470.
46 Sibille E, et al: GABA-related transcripts in the dorsolateral prefrontal cortex in mood disorders. Int J Neuropsychopharmacol 2011;14:721–734.
47 Tripp A, et al: Reduced somatostatin in subgenual anterior cingulate cortex in major depression. Neurobiol Dis 2011;42:116–124.
48 Tripp A, et al: Brain-derived neurotrophic factor signaling and subgenual anterior cingulate cortex dysfunction in major depressive disorder. Am J Psychiatry 2012;169:1194–1202.
49 Guilloux JP, et al: Molecular evidence for BDNF- and GABA-related dysfunctions in the amygdala of female subjects with major depression. Mol Psychiatry 2012;17:1130–1142.
50 Martel G, et al: Somatostatinergic systems: an update on brain functions in normal and pathological aging. Front Endocrinol (Lausanne) 2012;3:154.
51 Karolewicz B, et al: Reduced level of glutamic acid decarboxylase-67 kDa in the prefrontal cortex in major depression. Int J Neuropsychopharmacol 2010; 13:411–420.
52 Hasler G, et al: Reduced prefrontal glutamate/glutamine and gamma-aminobutyric acid levels in major depression determined using proton magnetic resonance spectroscopy. Arch Gen Psychiatry 2007;64: 193–200.
53 Levinson AJ, et al: Evidence of cortical inhibitory deficits in major depressive disorder. Biol Psychiatry 2010;67:458–464.
54 Gabbay V, et al: Anterior cingulate cortex gamma-aminobutyric acid in depressed adolescents: relationship to anhedonia. Arch Gen Psychiatry 2012;69: 139–149.
55 Hasler G, Northoff G: Discovering imaging endophenotypes for major depression. Mol Psychiatry 2011;16:604–619.
56 Sanacora G, et al: Increased occipital cortex GABA concentrations in depressed patients after therapy with selective serotonin reuptake inhibitors. Am J Psychiatry 2002;159:663–665.
57 Sanacora G, et al: Increased cortical GABA concentrations in depressed patients receiving ECT. Am J Psychiatry 2003;160:577–579.
58 Northoff G, et al: GABA concentrations in the human anterior cingulate cortex predict negative BOLD responses in fMRI. Nat Neurosci 2007;10: 1515–1517.
59 Brambilla P, et al: GABAergic dysfunction in mood disorders. Mol Psychiatry 2003;8:721–737, 715.
60 Luscher B, Shen Q, Sahir N: The GABAergic deficit hypothesis of major depressive disorder. Mol Psychiatry 2011;16:383–406.
61 Emrich HM, et al: Effect of sodium valproate on mania. The GABA-hypothesis of affective disorders. Arch Psychiatr Nervenkr 1980;229:1–16.
62 Gold BI, et al: GABA levels in CSF of patients with psychiatric disorders. Am J Psychiatry 1980;137: 362–364.
63 Petty F, Schlesser MA: Plasma GABA in affective illness. A preliminary investigation. J Affect Disord 1981;3:339–343.
64 Petty F, Sherman AD: Plasma GABA levels in psychiatric illness. J Affect Disord 1984;6:131–138.
65 Gerner RH, Hare TA: CSF GABA in normal subjects and patients with depression, schizophrenia, mania, and anorexia nervosa. Am J Psychiatry 1981;138: 1098–1101.
66 Earnheart JC, et al: GABAergic control of adult hippocampal neurogenesis in relation to behavior indicative of trait anxiety and depression states. J Neurosci 2007;27:3845–3854.
67 Mayberg HS, et al: Deep brain stimulation for treatment-resistant depression. Neuron 2005;45:651–660.
68 Morris HM, Hashimoto T, Lewis DA: Alterations in somatostatin mRNA expression in the dorsolateral prefrontal cortex of subjects with schizophrenia or schizoaffective disorder. Cereb Cortex 2008;18: 1575–1587.
69 Konradi C, et al: Hippocampal interneurons in bipolar disorder. Arch Gen Psychiatry 2011;68:340–350.
70 Konradi C, et al: Molecular evidence for mitochondrial dysfunction in bipolar disorder. Arch Gen Psychiatry 2004;61:300–308.
71 Timmers HJ, et al: Somatostatin 1–12 immunoreactivity is decreased in the hypothalamic lateral tuberal nucleus of Huntington's disease patients. Brain Res 1996;728:141–148.
72 Davies P, Katzman R, Terry RD: Reduced somatostatin-like immunoreactivity in cerebral cortex from cases of Alzheimer disease and Alzheimer senile dementia. Nature 1980;288:279–280.
73 Epelbaum J, et al: Somatostatin, Alzheimer's disease and cognition: an old story coming of age? Prog Neurobiol 2009;89:153–161.
74 Epelbaum J, et al: Somatostatin receptors in brain and pituitary. Horm Res 1989;31:45–50.
75 Lin LC, Sibille E: Reduced brain somatostatin in mood disorders: a common pathophysiological substrate and drug target? Front Pharmacol 2013;4:110.
76 Lin LC, Sibille E: Somatostatin, neuronal vulnerability and behavioral emotionality. Mol Psychiatry 2015;20:377–387.

77 Dwivedi Y: Brain-derived neurotrophic factor in suicide pathophysiology; in Dwivedi Y (ed): The Neurobiological Basis of Suicide. Boca Raton, CRC Press, 2012.
78 Pandey GN, et al: Brain-derived neurotrophic factor and tyrosine kinase B receptor signalling in postmortem brain of teenage suicide victims. Int J Neuropsychopharmacol 2008;11:1047–1061.
79 Dwivedi Y, et al: Altered gene expression of brain-derived neurotrophic factor and receptor tyrosine kinase B in postmortem brain of suicide subjects. Arch Gen Psychiatry 2003;60:804–815.
80 Keller S, et al: Increased BDNF promoter methylation in the Wernicke area of suicide subjects. Arch Gen Psychiatry 2010;67:258–267.
81 Perroud N, et al: Interaction between BDNF Val66Met and childhood trauma on adult's violent suicide attempt. Genes Brain Behav 2008;7:314–322.
82 Pregelj P, et al: The association between brain-derived neurotrophic factor polymorphism (BDNF Val66Met) and suicide. J Affect Disord 2011;128: 287–290.
83 Deltheil T, et al: Synergistic neurochemical and behavioural effects of acute intrahippocampal injection of brain-derived neurotrophic factor and antidepressants in adult mice. Int J Neuropsychopharmacol 2009;12:905–915.
84 Shirayama Y, et al: Brain-derived neurotrophic factor produces antidepressant effects in behavioral models of depression. J Neurosci 2002;22:3251–3261.
85 Karege F, et al: Neurotrophin levels in postmortem brains of suicide victims and the effects of antemortem diagnosis and psychotropic drugs. Brain Res Mol Brain Res 2005;136:29–37.
86 Block SG, Nemeroff CB: Emerging antidepressants to treat major depressive disorder. Asian J Psychiatr 2014;12:7–16.
87 Bersani FS, et al: Deep transcranial magnetic stimulation as a treatment for psychiatric disorders: a comprehensive review. Eur Psychiatry 2013;28:30–39.
88 Sher L, Mindes J, Novakovic V: Transcranial magnetic stimulation and the treatment of suicidality. Expert Rev Neurother 2010;10:1781–1784.
89 Desmyter S, et al: The acute effects of accelerated repetitive transcranial magnetic stimulation on suicide risk in unipolar depression: preliminary results. Psychiatr Danub 2014;26(suppl 1):48–52.
90 Rapinesi C, et al: Alcohol and suicidality: could deep transcranial magnetic stimulation (dTMS) be a possible treatment? Psychiatr Danub 2014;26: 281–284.
91 Hadley D, et al: Safety, tolerability, and effectiveness of high doses of adjunctive daily left prefrontal repetitive transcranial magnetic stimulation for treatment-resistant depression in a clinical setting. J ECT 2011;27:18–25.
92 George MS, et al: A two-site pilot randomized 3 day trial of high dose left prefrontal repetitive transcranial magnetic stimulation (rTMS) for suicidal inpatients. Brain Stimul 2014;7:421–431.
93 Padberg F, George MS: Repetitive transcranial magnetic stimulation of the prefrontal cortex in depression. Exp Neurol 2009;219:2–13.
94 O'Reardon JP, et al: Efficacy and safety of transcranial magnetic stimulation in the acute treatment of major depression: a multisite randomized controlled trial. Biol Psychiatry 2007;62:1208–1216.
95 Kujirai T, et al: Corticocortical inhibition in human motor cortex. J Physiol 1993;471:501–519.
96 Cantello R, et al: Magnetic brain stimulation: the silent period after the motor evoked potential. Neurology 1992;42:1951–1959.
97 Siebner HR, et al: Continuous intrathecal baclofen infusions induced a marked increase of the transcranially evoked silent period in a patient with generalized dystonia. Muscle Nerve 1998;21:1209–1212.
98 Ziemann U, et al: Effects of antiepileptic drugs on motor cortex excitability in humans: a transcranial magnetic stimulation study. Ann Neurol 1996;40: 367–378.
99 Thompson SM, Gahwiler BH: Effects of the GABA uptake inhibitor tiagabine on inhibitory synaptic potentials in rat hippocampal slice cultures. J Neurophysiol 1992;67:1698–1701.
100 de Jesus DR, et al: Determining optimal rTMS parameters through changes in cortical inhibition. Clin Neurophysiol 2014;125:755–762.
101 Daskalakis ZJ, et al: The effects of repetitive transcranial magnetic stimulation on cortical inhibition in healthy human subjects. Exp Brain Res 2006;174: 403–412.

Dr. Etienne Sibille
Neurobiology of Depression and Aging, Campbell Family Mental Health Research Institute
Centre for Addiction and Mental Health, Room 134, University of Toronto
250 College Street
Toronto, ON M5T 1R8 (Canada)
E-Mail Etienne.Sibille@camh.ca

Kaschka WP, Rujescu D (eds): Biological Aspects of Suicidal Behavior.
Adv Biol Psychiatry. Basel, Karger, 2016, vol 30, pp 51–62 (DOI: 10.1159/000438468)

Genetics of Suicidal Behavior

Ina Giegling · Dan Rujescu

Department of Psychiatry, Psychotherapy and Psychosomatics, Martin Luther University Halle-Wittenberg, Halle, Germany

Abstract

Suicidal behavior is multidimensional. As well as medical, psychological, psychosocial, social, cultural, and socioeconomic parameters, it also includes biological, especially genetic, risk factors. The heritability is about 55% assuming a polygenic risk model. First linkage and candidate gene studies have focused mainly on the serotonergic system. Interestingly, most associations were found not with suicidal behavior per se but with personality traits like aggression and impulsivity. Newly started genome-wide association studies are promising but actually mostly do not show genome-wide significant results. The main reason seems to lie in the sample size. Exome and whole genome sequencing studies are in their earliest beginnings and will hopefully help to dissect the genetic risk proportion of suicidal behavior.

Heritability of Suicidal Behavior

Someone commits suicide worldwide every 40 s. This makes over 1 million people each year. The number of suicide attempts is 10-fold higher. Suicide accounts for 2% of the world's death. It has emerged as one of the leading causes of death among adolescents. Suicide is the second leading cause of death among 15- to 29-year-olds [1]. Attempted suicide is regarded as the most important predictor of a future death from suicide [2]. Almost one quarter of suicides are preceded by nonfatal suicidal behavior in the previous year [3]. Nearly 2% of suicide attempters end their own life during the 12 months subsequent to the index event [4].

Suicidal behavior is complex and mostly a consequence of interactions of risk factors like medical (e.g. mental disorders), psychological (e.g. hopelessness, impulsivity, aggression), psychosocial (e.g. social isolation), social (e.g. lack of social support), cultural (e.g. religion), socioeconomic (e.g. unemployment), and biological factors (e.g. genetics, disorders in brain functioning) [5]. The genetic risk is supported by family, twin and adoption studies, indicating that suicidal acts have a genetic contribution that is independent of the heritability of psychopathology [6, 7].

One of the largest epidemiological studies by Mittendorfer-Rutz et al. [8] including 14,440 suicide attempters and 144,440 healthy controls showed that the risk of suicide attempts increased by a factor of 4.2 when the biological mother had committed a suicide attempt or by a factor of 3.3 when the father was affected. Furthermore, the risk was increased by 4.5 when siblings showed suicidal behavior or by a factor of 3.7 if any family member was involved. If suicide attempts were present in 2 or more family members the risk for an own suicide attempt increased by a factor of 7.3 [8]. This familial accumulation of suicidal behavior could be partly due to genetic risk factors. Twin studies compare the concordance for suicidal behavior in monozygotic twins, which mostly share 100% of their genes, with dizygotic twins sharing 50% of them. This allows us to separate effects due to a shared environment from genetic factors. Roy et al. [9] examined 62 monozygotic and 114 dizygotic twin pairs and reported concordance rates of 11.3 and 1.8%, respectively. An Australian twin study with a total of nearly 6,000 twins estimated the heritability of suicide attempts at 55% [10]. Interestingly, Voracek and Loibl [11] found convergent evidence from a multitude of research designs (adoption, family, genome scan, geographical, immigrant, molecular genetics, surname, and twin studies of suicide) suggesting genetic contributions to suicide risk. Their work focused on twin studies. A total of 32 studies located through extensive literature search strategies were analyzed (19 case reports, 5 twin register-based studies, 4 population-based epidemiological studies, 4 studies of surviving co-twins). The literature was based on publications between 1812 and 2006 in six languages and reports data from 13 countries. A meta-analysis of all register-based studies and all case reports aggregated showed that concordance for completed suicide was significantly more frequent among monozygotic (24.1%) than dizygotic twin pairs (2.3%). The totality of evidence from twin studies of suicide strongly suggests genetic contributions to liability for suicidal behavior [11]. Adoption studies have been less commonly performed and classical studies often used the same Danish health statistics register [12–14]. The investigation of Schulsinger [13] identified 57 suicide victims among early adopted Danish citizens and defined them as index cases. The biological relatives of these index cases showed a 6-fold higher suicide rate (4.46%) than the biological relatives of a matched, nonsuicidal adoptee control group (0.74%). Furthermore, there was no suicide among the adoptive relatives of the index cases. von Borczyskowski et al. [15] presented a very large study based on the Swedish registry with a total of 2,471,496 people, including 27,600 adoptees, supporting the role of a genetic risk.

Association Studies of Suicidal Behavior

Serotonergic System

The involvement of serotonin in suicidal behavior is already known since the 70s. Clinical studies found lower levels of the serotonin metabolite 5-hydroxyindoleacetic acid (5-HIAA), a putative indicator for low serotonin turnover, in suicidal patients [16, 17]. Furthermore, many studies investigating postmortem brains of suicide victims have shown alterations of the serotonergic system, especially in the prefrontal cortex [18]. Besides that, low CSF 5-HIAA is associated with aggressiveness, low social affiliation, high-risk behavior, and premature mortality [19, 20]. In humans, 5-HIAA in the CSF correlates inversely with various aggressive behaviors, as demonstrated in healthy and psychiatric samples throughout the life span. Most genetic association studies have focused on genes involved in serotonergic neurotransmission. Serotonergic function was regarded as crucial for the regulation of impulsive and aggressive behavior, which in turn has been demonstrated to correlate with suicidal behavior in various studies [21].

Tryptophan Hydroxylases 1

Serotonin (5-hydroxytryptamine, 5-HT) is a monoamine neurotransmitter. Biochemically, L-Tryptophan is converted to 5-hydroxy-L-tryptophan through tryptophan hydroxylase (TPH). This enzyme is a rate-limiting step to 5-hydroxytryptophan. To find genetic risk factors for suicidal behavior, early studies concentrated on single nucleotide polymorphisms (SNPs) in these genes. A first meta-analysis [22] did not find an association of the commonly studied intron 7 A218C (TPH1) SNP with suicidal behavior per se. A further meta-analysis summarized the results of 7 studies investigating the A218C SNP in Caucasians and found a higher frequency of the A218 allele in patients [23]. Another meta-analysis including 9 studies confirmed the association for the A218C polymorphism [24]. Li et al. [25] provided a meta-analysis of 22 studies and showed further support for association. Additional support for the involvement of THP1 (SNP rs1800532) and suicidal behavior was provided by the meta-analysis by Clayden et al. [26].

Recently, a meta-analysis was conducted with a total of 37 genetic association studies of TPH1 (A218C and A779C). Subgroup analyses were done by Caucasian and Asian populations. In the case of TPH1 gene variants (A218C and A779C), 5,683 cases and 11,652 controls were involved. The analyses provided evidence that A218C/A779C TPH1 variants may be risk factors for the presentation of suicidal behavior, which is in agreement with previously reported meta-analyses [27].

Interestingly, this risk allele 'A' was also associated with aggression and anger [28]. This result was further supported by Rujescu et al. [29], who showed that A carriers had higher scores on the Trait Anger Scale of the STAXI (State Trait Anger Expression Inventory) in 2 independent samples (healthy controls and suicide attempters). An involvement of TPH1 in anger and aggression phenotypes was furthermore presented by Baud et al. [30], who reported that suicide attempters carrying the AA genotype scored significantly lower on the anger control subscale than C allele carriers. A number of further studies showed the involvement of TPH1 in personality traits. For example, Cicchetti et al. [31] explored the hypothesis that TPH1 interacted with maltreatment subtype to predict peer reports of antisocial behavior. TPH1 polymorphisms also moderated the effects of maltreatment subtype on adult reports of antisocial behavior; genetic effects were strongest for children who were abused. Additionally, TPH1 moderated the effect of developmental timing of maltreatment and chronicity on adult reports of antisocial behavior [31]. Andre et al. [32] reported that the number of TPH1 A alleles was associated with increasing levels in novelty seeking (NS) scores 1 and 2 and decreasing levels in harm avoidance (HA) 1 and 2 between TPH1 A218C genotypes. TPH1 genotype and treatment response had an interactive effect on both HA1 and HA2 and to a lesser degree on NS2 scores. Additionally, an interaction between remission status and TPH1 A218C genotype was found to be associated with the end point HA score, with a more marked effect of the interaction between the CC genotype and remission status compared to A allele carriers [32].

Tryptophan Hydroxylases 2

Walther et al. [33] discovered a second TPH isoform in mice – termed TPH2 [34]. Breidenthal et al. [35] screened the coding and exon-flanking intronic sequence of the TPH2 gene and identified several genetic variants that might serve as markers for association studies. The investigation of SNPs in the TPH2 gene in a sample of suicide victims and matched controls showed an association of one SNP with completed suicide [36]. Since then several case-control studies have been provided showing positive and negative results (for review, see Tsai et al. [37]). Lately, a meta-analysis by Gonzales-Castro et al. [27] analyzed three TPH2 SNPs (G-703 T, A-473 T and G19918A) in 4,196 cases and 5,990 controls. The meta-analysis did not detect any significant association with patients presenting suicidal behavior for these variants [27]. In addition, Choong et al. [38] provided a meta-analysis on 2,536 cases and 3,101 controls for nine TPH2 SNPs (rs4570625, rs7305115, rs1386486, rs11178997, rs1386493, rs1386494, rs1386495, rs10784941, and rs4290270) based on 11 case-control studies with 13 independent samples published between 1998 and 2013. No significant results were detected, suggesting that TPH2 may not play a significant role in suicidal behavior per se.

Interestingly, polymorphisms in the TPH2 gene were associated with personality traits like aggression or impulsivity [39–41], cognitive control and emotion regulation [42] and neuroticism [43, 44] but more studies including large sample sizes are necessary to provide further support.

Serotonin Transporter

The serotonin transporter (5-HTT) is responsible for the reuptake of released serotonin from the synaptic cleft. The 5′-promotor region of the 5-HTT gene contains a functional insertion/deletion variant (5-HTTLPR) with former 2 and later 3 common alleles that were designated as 'short' (s) and 'long' (l_A and l_G). A meta-analysis conducted by Anguelova et al. [45] included 12 studies investigating the 5-HTT promoter polymorphism. The study samples compromised 10 Caucasian populations, 1 US population and 1 Chinese sample. There was a total number of 1,168 cases (suicide completers and suicide attempters) and 1,371 controls. A significant association was found with the s allele and suicidal behavior. A following meta-analysis, including 18 studies with 1,521 suicide attempters or completers and 2,429 controls, found no association [46]. Interestingly, they observed an association of the s allele with violent suicidal behavior. Three years later Li and He [47] provided a meta-analysis including 39 studies and examined the association between suicide attempts and the s allele. Clayden et al. [26] analyzed the association between the serotonin transporter s allele and suicidal behavior in 31 primary case-control studies (6,324 cases, 10,285 controls) with no significance. When only the attempted suicide case-control studies were analyzed, the pooled OR reached significance. A recent meta-analysis by Schild et al. [48], including 2,536 cases and 3,984 controls, further supports the involvement of the 5-HTTLPR in suicidal behavior. More detailed studies are required, as it seems that this functional variant is associated with particular intermediate phenotypes of suicidal behavior [for review, see 49–51].

Serotonin Receptors

There are several serotonin receptors named from 5-HT_1 to 5-HT_7, including various subtypes. For the most part, the following genes for serotonin receptors were analyzed in the context of suicidal behavior.

5-HT_{1A} Receptor

Lemonde et al. [52] examined the common C-1019G SNP in the promoter region in a sample of suicide victims and controls. They found the G allele to be significantly overrepresented in the suicide group. This association was not replicated by Huang et al. [53]. The investigation of the structural polymorphisms Pro16Leu and Gly272Asp revealed no association with suicidal behavior in Japanese subjects [54] and the result for the Pro16Leu was replicated by a second Japanese group [55]. A meta-analysis for the A6526G polymorphism provided no association [25] and three further meta-analyses for the C1019G variant showed no significance [26, 48, 56].

5-HT_{1B} Receptor

Genetic variants within the 5-HT_{1B} gene seem not to play a crucial role in suicidal behavior. Kia-Keating et al. [57] performed a meta-analysis on 789 cases and 1,247 controls with negative results. Furthermore, Clayden et al. [26] including 2,948 cases and 4,066 controls and Schild et al. [48] with 1,161 cases and 1,826 controls did not provide evidence for association. However, there seems to be an association with aggressive behavior. Studies of serotonin 1B knockout mice show an increase in aggressive behavior relative to wild-type mice [58]. Interestingly, Jensen et al. [59] provided evidence that a common polymorphism moderates regulation by miR-96 and associates with aggressive human behaviors. Furthermore, Conner et al. [60] showed that functional polymorphisms predict self-reported anger and hostility among young men. Recently, Hakulinen et al. [61] examined whether HTR1B is related to hostility, anger and aggressive behavior phenotypes over a lifespan and whether it modifies the connection between childhood aggressive behavior and adulthood hostility and anger. The participants were 967 women and men from a large population-based sample (the Young Finns Study) with a 27-year follow-up. HTR1B SNP rs6296 was associated with childhood aggressive behavior but not with adulthood anger or hostility and modified the association between childhood aggressive behavior and adulthood hostility [61].

5-HT_{2A} Receptor

The 5-HT_{2A} receptor gene has been regarded as a major candidate for genetic susceptibility due to the increased density of brain and platelet serotonin 2A (5-HT_{2A}) receptors in subjects with suicidal behavior [62]. However, a first meta-analysis pooling 9 studies with 596 suicide completers or attempters and 1,003 controls did not find any association with the T102C SNP [45]. A later meta-analysis of 25 studies supported this result and more recent meta-analyses also did not provide an association of this SNP [25, 26, 48], including the latest by Wang et al. [63]. Interestingly, a meta-analysis with another genetic variant within the promoter (A1438G; rs20070040) showed an association [64]. This same SNP was also associated with major depressive disorder (MDD) in a recent meta-analysis including 9 studies with a total of 1,510 patients and 2,281 controls. The study suggests that the A allele of the A1438G polymorphism might play a role in susceptibility to MDD. On the contrary, the T102C polymorphism does not seem to be capable of modifying MDD risk [65].

Dopaminergic System and Catecholamines

CSF studies provided support for the involvement of dopamine in suicidal behavior, showing correlations between low levels of the dopamine metabolite homovanillic acid and suicidal behavior [66]. The following will only mention genetic association where meta-analyses with a sufficient number of studies are available.

Catechol-O-Methyltransferase

Catechol-O-Methyltransferase (COMT) is a major enzyme involved in the inactivation of the catecholamines dopamine and noradrenalin. The functional polymorphism replacing valine (Val) at codon 158 with methionine (Met) was studied intensively in psychiatric diseases by Lachman et al. [67].

For suicidal behavior Kia-Keating et al. [57] provided a meta-analysis based on 6 related studies including 519 cases and 933 control subjects. There was evidence of a significant association between the COMT 158 Met polymorphism and suicidal behavior. The meta-analysis by Calati et al. [68] included 10 studies with 1,324 patients and found no association. Further meta-analyses also provided no significance [26, 48, 69].

Further Genes

Brain-Derived Neurotrophic Factor

A high number of further genes have been studied in the context of suicidal behavior. Brain-derived neurotrophic factor (BDNF) should be mentioned as an example. BDNF is a member of the neurotrophin family of growth factors. The first meta-analysis was performed by Zai et al. [70], who performed an analysis of the functional BDNF marker $Val^{66}Met$ (rs6265, 196G>A) in suicidal behavior using data from 11 previously published samples plus their own sample (total n = 3,352 subjects, 1,202 with history of suicidal behavior). The meta-analysis showed a trend for the Met-carrying genotypes and the Met allele conferring risk for suicide. Furthermore, they found the Met allele and the Met allele-carrying genotypes associated with history of suicide attempt (8 studies).

Genome-Wide Association Studies of Suicidal Behavior

The last years have provided a new stage of technical possibilities in genetic association studies. More than one million SNPs were studied in parallel and also first exome or whole genome sequencing studies are under way. Up to now only a few of these studies have been looking at suicidal behavior.

Treatment-Emergent Suicidal Ideation

Laje et al. [71] performed a genome-wide association study (GWAS) on treatment-emergent suicidal ideation (TESI). A clinically representative cohort of outpatients with nonpsychotic MDD enrolled in the Sequenced Treatment Alternatives to Relieve Depression (STAR*D) trial were treated with citalopram under a standard protocol for up to 14 weeks. DNA samples from 90 white participants who developed TESI and a sex-matched and race-matched equal number of treated participants who denied any suicidal ideas were genotyped with 109,365 SNPs on the Illumina Human-1 BeadChip (Illumina, San Diego, Calif., USA). One SNP in PAPLN was genome-wide significant and another SNP in IL28RA showed a trend. Another TESI study was provided by Perroud et al. [72]. A total of 706 patients treated for major depression with escitalopram or nortriptyline over 12 weeks in the Genome-Based Therapeutic Drugs for Depression (GENDEP) study were genotyped with Illumina Human 610-Quad BeadChips. A total of 244 subjects experienced an increase in suicidal ideation during follow-up. The genetic marker most significantly associated with increasing suicidality was an SNP (rs11143230) located 30 kb downstream of a gene encoding guanine deaminase (GDA) on chromosome 9q21.13.

A third GWAS on TESI within the MARS study was provided by Menke et al. [73]. The study was evaluated in depressed inpatients (n = 397) and defined by an emergence of suicidal thoughts during hospitalization without suicidal thoughts at admission using the suicide item 3 of the Hamilton Depression Rating Scale. Genotype distribution of 405,383 SNPs in patients with TESI (n = 32, 8.1%) was compared to patients without an increase in suicidal ideation (n = 329, 82.9%) and to a subgroup who never reported suicidal ideation (n = 79, 19.9%). Top results were analyzed in an independent sample (n = 501). No variant reached genome-wide significance.

Suicide Attempts

Perlis et al. [74] provided the first GWAS on suicide attempts. The authors analyzed data on lifetime suicide attempts from GWAS of bipolar I and II disorder as well as MDD. The strongest evidence of association for suicide attempt in bipolar disorder was observed in a region without identified genes (rs1466846); five loci also showed suggestive evidence of association. In major depression, the strongest evidence of association was observed for an SNP in ABI3BP, with six loci also showing suggestive association.

One year later Schosser et al. [75] presented a genome-wide association scan of suicidal thoughts and behavior in major depression. No SNP was associated at genome-wide significance level. For the quantitative trait, evidence of association was detected at GFRA1, a receptor for the neurotrophin GDRA. For the discrete trait of suicide attempt, SNPs in KIAA1244 and RGS18 showed trends. None of these SNPs showed evidence for replication in the additional cohorts tested. Candidate gene analyses provided some support for a polymorphism in NTRK2, which was previously associated with suicidality. Willour et al. [76] conducted an attempted suicide GWAS that compared the genotypes of 1,201 bipolar patients with a history of suicide attempts to the genotypes of 1,497 bipolar patients without a history of suicidal behavior. None of these SNPs were significantly associated in the replication sample after correcting for multiple testing but the combined analysis of the 2 sample sets produced an association signal on 2p25 (rs300774) at the threshold of genome-wide significance. The associated SNPs on 2p25 fall in a large linkage disequilibrium block containing the ACP1 (acid phosphatase 1) gene, a gene whose expression is significantly elevated in bipolar patients who have completed suicide. Furthermore, the ACP1 protein is a tyrosine phosphatase that influences Wnt signaling, a pathway regulated by lithium, making ACP1 a functional candidate for involvement in the phenotype [76].

Based on the previous GENDEP study, Mullins et al. [77] derived polygenic scores from each sample and tested their ability to predict suicide attempts in the mood disorder cohorts or ideation status in the GENDEP study. Polygenic scores for MDD, bipolar disorder and schizophrenia from the Psychiatric Genomics Consortium were used to investigate pleiotropy between psychiatric disorders and suicide phenotypes. No significant evidence for association was detected at any SNP in the GWAS or meta-analysis. Polygenic scores for MDD significantly predicted suicidal ideation in the GENDEP pharmacogenetics study and also predicted suicidal behavior in a combined validation data set. Polygenic scores for suicidal behavior showed no predictive ability for suicidal ideation [77]. A recent SNP GWAS on suicidal behavior was published by Zai et al. [78], who conducted a GWAS of suicide behavior severity in 3 independent samples of bipolar patients: 212 small nuclear families with bipolar patients, a further 428 patients and 483 patients from the UK. No genome-wide significant association of any tested markers in any of the bipolar samples was detected [78]. The latest GWAS on suicidal behavior was performed by Galfalvy et al. [79]. A consortium of US, Canadian and German teams assembled 2 groups of cases: suicide attempters and suicides (n = 577) and nonattempter psychiatric and healthy controls (n = 1,233). Logistic regression was used to test for association. The test was repeated separating suicide attempt and completed suicide as outcomes. No SNP reached genome-wide significance but several SNPs within STK3 (neuronal cell death), ADAMTS14, PSME2 (both linked to inflammatory response), and TBX20 (brainstem motor neuron development) genes reached $p < 1 \times 10^{-5}$. Pathway analysis identified the following pathways: 'cellular assembly and organization', 'nervous system development and function', 'cell death and survival', 'immunological disease', 'infectious disease', and 'inflammatory response' [79].

In summary, GWAS have only started and a greater number of larger samples need to be combined to make valid conclusions. There is hope that new exome and whole genome sequencing studies will contribute to our knowledge of genetic risk factors for suicidal behavior.

References

1 WHO. World Health Report. Health Systems. WHO, Geneva. www.who.int.

2 Beghi M, Rosenbaum JF, Cerri C, Cornaggia CM: Risk factors for fatal and nonfatal repetition of suicide attempts: a literature review. Neuropsychiatr Dis Treat 2013;9:1725–1736.

3 Owens D, House A: General hospital services for deliberate self-harm. Haphazard clinical provision, little research, no central strategy. J R Coll Physicians Lond 1994;28:370–371.

4 Owens D, Horrocks J, House A: Fatal and non-fatal repetition of self-harm. Systematic review. Br J Psychiatry 2002;181:193–199.

5 Wasserman D, Wasserman C: The Oxford Textbook of Suicidology and Suicide Prevention: A Global Perspective. Oxford, Oxford University Press, 2009.

6 Brent DA, Mann JJ: Family genetic studies, suicide, and suicidal behavior. Am J Med Genet C Semin Med Genet 2005;133C:13–24.

7 Turecki G: The molecular bases of the suicidal brain. Nat Rev Neurosci 2014;15:802–816.

8 Mittendorfer-Rutz E, Rasmussen F, Wasserman D: Familial clustering of suicidal behaviour and psychopathology in young suicide attempters. A register-based nested case control study. Soc Psychiatry Psychiatr Epidemiol 2008;43:28–36.

9 Roy A, Segal NL, Centerwall BS, Robinette CD: Suicide in twins. Arch Gen Psychiatry 1991;48:29–32.

10 Statham DJ, Heath AC, Madden PA, Bucholz KK, Bierut L, Dinwiddie SH, Slutske WS, Dunne MP, Martin NG: Suicidal behaviour: an epidemiological and genetic study. Psychol Med 1998;28:839–855.

11 Voracek M, Loibl LM: Genetics of suicide: a systematic review of twin studies. Wien Klin Wochenschr 2007;119:463–475.

12 Kety SS: Biochemistry and mental states. Calif Med 1968;108:362–368.

13 Schulsinger F: A family study of suicide; in Schov M, Stromgren G (eds): Origin, Prevention and Treatment of Affective Disorders. London/New York, Academic Press, 1979, pp 277–287.

14 Wender PH, Kety SS, Rosenthal D, Schulsinger F, Ortmann J, Lunde I: Psychiatric disorders in the biological and adoptive families of adopted individuals with affective disorders. Arch Gen Psychiatry 1986; 43:923–929.
15 von Borczyskowski A, Lindblad F, Vinnerljung B, Reintjes R, Hjern A: Familial factors and suicide: an adoption study in a Swedish National Cohort. Psychol Med 2011;41:749–758.
16 Asberg M, Traskman L, Thoren P: 5-HIAA in the cerebrospinal fluid. A biochemical suicide predictor? Arch Gen Psychiatry 1976;33:1193–1197.
17 Asberg M: Neurotransmitters and suicidal behavior. The evidence from cerebrospinal fluid studies. Ann N Y Acad Sci 1997;836:158–181.
18 Arango V, Underwood MD, Mann JJ: Postmortem findings in suicide victims. Implications for in vivo imaging studies. Ann N Y Acad Sci 1997;836:269–287.
19 Higley JD, Mehlman PT, Poland RE, Taub DM, Vickers J, Suomi SJ, Linnoila M: CSF testosterone and 5-HIAA correlate with different types of aggressive behaviors. Biol Psychiatry 1996a;40:1067–1082.
20 Mehlman PT, Higley JD, Faucher I, Lilly AA, Taub DM, Vickers J, Suomi SJ, Linnoila M: Low CSF 5-HIAA concentrations and severe aggression and impaired impulse control in nonhuman primates. Am J Psychiatry 1994;151:1485–1491.
21 Mann JJ: Neurobiology of suicidal behaviour. Nat Rev Neurosci 2003;4:819–828.
22 Lalovic A, Turecki G: Meta-analysis of the association between tryptophan hydroxylase and suicidal behavior. Am J Med Genet 2002;114:533–540.
23 Rujescu D, Giegling I, Sato T, Hartmann AM, Moller HJ: Genetic variations in tryptophan hydroxylase in suicidal behavior: analysis and meta-analysis. Biol Psychiatry 2003;54:465–473.
24 Bellivier F, Chaste P, Malafosse A: Association between the TPH gene A218C polymorphism and suicidal behavior: a meta-analysis. Am J Med Genet B Neuropsychiatr Genet 2004;124B:87–91.
25 Li D, Duan Y, He L: Association study of serotonin 2A receptor (5-HT_{2A}) gene with schizophrenia and suicidal behavior using systematic meta-analysis. Biochem Biophys Res Commun 2006;340:1006–1015.
26 Clayden RC, Zaruk A, Meyre D, Thabane L, Samaan Z: The association of attempted suicide with genetic variants in the SLC6A4 and TPH genes depends on the definition of suicidal behavior: a systematic review and meta-analysis. Transl Psychiatry 2012;2: e166.
27 González-Castro TB, Juárez-Rojop I, López-Narváez ML, Tovilla-Zárate CA: Association of TPH-1 and TPH-2 gene polymorphisms with suicidal behavior: a systematic review and meta-analysis. BMC Psychiatry 2014;14:196.
28 Manuck SB, Flory JD, Ferrell RE, Dent KM, Mann JJ, Muldoon MF: Aggression and anger-related traits associated with a polymorphism of the tryptophan hydroxylase gene. Biol Psychiatry 1999;45:603–614.
29 Rujescu D, Giegling I, Bondy B, Gietl A, Zill P, Moller HJ: Association of anger-related traits with SNPs in the TPH gene. Mol Psychiatry 2002;7:1023–1029.
30 Baud P, Perroud N, Courtet P, Jaussent I, Relecom C, Jollant F, Malafosse A: Modulation of anger control in suicide attempters by TPH-1. Genes Brain Behav 2009;8:97–100.
31 Cicchetti D, Rogosch FA, Thibodeau EL: The effects of child maltreatment on early signs of antisocial behavior: genetic moderation by tryptophan hydroxylase, serotonin transporter, and monoamine oxidase A genes. Dev Psychopathol 2012;24:907–928.
32 Andre K, Kampman O, Viikki M, Illi A, Setälä-Soikkeli E, Poutanen O, Mononen N, Leinonen E, Lehtimäki T: TPH1 A218C polymorphism and temperament in major depression. BMC Psychiatry 2013;13:118.
33 Walther DJ, Peter JU, Bashammakh S, Hortnagl H, Voits M, Fink H, Bader M: Synthesis of serotonin by a second tryptophan hydroxylase isoform. Science 2003;299:76.
34 Zhang X, Beaulieu JM, Sotnikova TD, Gainetdinov RR, Caron MG: Tryptophan hydroxylase-2 controls brain serotonin synthesis. Science 2004;305:217.
35 Breidenthal SE, White DJ, Glatt CE: Identification of genetic variants in the neuronal form of tryptophan hydroxylase (TPH2). Psychiatr Genet 2004;14:69–72.
36 Zill P, Buttner A, Eisenmenger W, Moller HJ, Bondy B, Ackenheil M: Single nucleotide polymorphism and haplotype analysis of a novel tryptophan hydroxylase isoform (TPH2) gene in suicide victims. Biol Psychiatry 2004;56:581–586.
37 Tsai SJ, Hong CJ, Liou YJ: Recent molecular genetic studies and methodological issues in suicide research. Prog Neuropsychopharmacol Biol Psychiatry 2011;35:809–817.
38 Choong MY, Tee SF, Tang PY: Meta-analysis of polymorphisms in TPH2 gene and suicidal behavior. Psychiatry Res 2014;220:1163–1166.
39 Kulikov AV, Osipova DV, Naumenko VS, Popova NK: The C1473G polymorphism in the tryptophan hydroxylase-2 gene and intermale aggression in mice. Dokl Biol Sci 2005a;402:208–210.
40 Osipova DV, Kulikov AV, Popova NK: C1473G polymorphism in mouse tph2 gene is linked to tryptophan hydroxylase-2 activity in the brain, intermale aggression, and depressive-like behavior in the forced swim test. J Neurosci Res 2009;87:1168–1174.
41 Yoon HK, Lee HJ, Kim L, Lee MS, Ham BJ: Impact of tryptophan hydroxylase 2 G-703T polymorphism on anger-related personality traits and orbitofrontal cortex. Behav Brain Res 2012;231:105–110.

42 Waider J, Araragi N, Gutknecht L, Lesch KP: Tryptophan hydroxylase-2 (TPH2) in disorders of cognitive control and emotion regulation: a perspective. Psychoneuroendocrinology 2011;36:393–405.
43 Hong KW, Weiss A, Morimura N, Udono T, Hayasaka I, Humle T, Murayama Y, Ito S, Inoue-Murayama M: Polymorphism of the tryptophan hydroxylase 2 (TPH2) gene is associated with chimpanzee neuroticism. PLoS One 2011;6:e22144.
44 Lehto K, Vaht M, Mäestu J, Veidebaum T, Harro J: Effect of tryptophan hydroxylase-2 gene polymorphism G-703 T on personality in a population representative sample. Prog Neuropsychopharmacol Biol Psychiatry 2015;57:31–35.
45 Anguelova M, Benkelfat C, Turecki G: A systematic review of association studies investigating genes coding for serotonin receptors and the serotonin transporter. II. Suicidal behavior. Mol Psychiatry 2003;8: 646–653.
46 Lin PY, Tsai G: Association between serotonin transporter gene promoter polymorphism and suicide: results of a meta-analysis. Biol Psychiatry 2004;55: 1023–1030.
47 Li D, He L: Meta-analysis supports association between serotonin transporter (5-HTT) and suicidal behavior. Mol Psychiatry 2007;12:47–54.
48 Schild AH, Pietschnig J, Tran US, Voracek M: Genetic association studies between SNPs and suicidal behavior: a meta-analytical field synopsis. Prog Neuropsychopharmacol Biol Psychiatry 2013;46:36–42.
49 Murphy DL, Lesch KP: Targeting the murine serotonin transporter: insights into human neurobiology. Nat Rev Neurosci 2008;9:85–96.
50 Lesch KP: Linking emotion to the social brain. The role of the serotonin transporter in human social behaviour. EMBO Rep 2007;8:S24–S29.
51 Canli T, Lesch KP: Long story short: the serotonin transporter in emotion regulation and social cognition. Nat Neurosci 2007;10:1103–1109.
52 Lemonde S, Turecki G, Bakish D, Du L, Hrdina PD, Bown CD, Sequeira A, Kushwaha N, Morris SJ, Basak A, Ou XM, Albert PR: Impaired repression at a 5-hydroxytryptamine 1A receptor gene polymorphism associated with major depression and suicide. J Neurosci 2003;23:8788–8799.
53 Huang YY, Battistuzzi C, Oquendo MA, Harkavy-Friedman J, Greenhill L, Zalsman G, Brodsky B, Arango V, Brent DA, Mann JJ: Human 5-HT_{1A} receptor C(−1019)G polymorphism and psychopathology. Int J Neuropsychopharmacol 2004;7:441–451.
54 Nishiguchi N, Shirakawa O, Ono H, Nishimura A, Nushida H, Ueno Y, Maeda K: Lack of an association between 5-HT_{1A} receptor gene structural polymorphisms and suicide victims. Am J Med Genet 2002; 114:423–425.
55 Ohtani M, Shindo S, Yoshioka N: Polymorphisms of the tryptophan hydroxylase gene and serotonin 1A receptor gene in suicide victims among Japanese. Tohoku J Exp Med 2004;202:123–133.
56 Angles MR, Ocaña DB, Medellín BC, Tovilla-Zárate C: No association between the HTR_{1A} gene and suicidal behavior: a meta-analysis. Rev Bras Psiquiatr 2012;34:38–42.
57 Kia-Keating BM, Glatt SJ, Tsuang MT: Meta-analyses suggest association between COMT, but not HTR1B, alleles, and suicidal behavior. Am J Med Genet B Neuropsychiatr Genet 2007;144B:1048–1053.
58 Saudou F, Amara DA, Dierich A, LeMeur M, Ramboz S, Segu L, Buhot MC, Hen R: Enhanced aggressive behavior in mice lacking 5-HT_{1B} receptor. Science 1994;265:1875–1878.
59 Jensen KP, Covault J, Conner TS, Tennen H, Kranzler HR, Furneaux HM: A common polymorphism in serotonin receptor 1B mRNA moderates regulation by miR-96 and associates with aggressive human behaviors. Mol Psychiatry 2009;14:381–389.
60 Conner TS, Jensen KP, Tennen H, Furneaux HM, Kranzler HR, Covault J: Functional polymorphisms in the serotonin 1B receptor gene (HTR1B) predict self-reported anger and hostility among young men. Am J Med Genet B Neuropsychiatr Genet 2010;153B: 67–78.
61 Hakulinen C, Jokela M, Hintsanen M, Merjonen P, Pulkki-Råback L, Seppälä I, Lyytikäinen LP, Lehtimäki T, Kähönen M, Viikari J, Raitakari OT, Keltikangas-Järvinen L: Serotonin receptor 1B genotype and hostility, anger and aggressive behavior through the lifespan: the Young Finns study. J Behav Med 2013;36:583–590.
62 Bachus SE, Hyde TM, Akil M, Weickert CS, Vawter MP, Kleinman JE: Neuropathology of suicide. A review and an approach. Ann N Y Acad Sci 1997;836: 201–219.
63 Wang JY, Jia CX, Lian Y, Sun SH, Lyu M, Wu A: Association of the HTR2A 102T/C polymorphism with attempted suicide: a meta-analysis. Psychiatr Genet 2015;25:168–177.
64 Li D, He L: Further clarification of the contribution of the tryptophan hydroxylase (TPH) gene to suicidal behavior using systematic allelic and genotypic meta-analyses. Hum Genet 2006;119:233–240.
65 Zhao X, Sun L, Sun YH, Ren C, Chen J, Wu ZQ, Jiang YH, Lv XL: Association of HTR2A T102C and A-1438G polymorphisms with susceptibility to major depressive disorder: a meta-analysis. Neurol Sci 2014;35:1857–1866.
66 Ryding E, Lindström M, Träskman-Bendz L: The role of dopamine and serotonin in suicidal behaviour and aggression. Prog Brain Res 2008;172:307–315.

67 Lachman HM, Papolos DF, Saito T, Yu YM, Szumlanski CL, Weinshilboum RM: Human catechol-O-methyltransferase pharmacogenetics: description of a functional polymorphism and its potential application to neuropsychiatric disorders. Pharmacogenetics 1996;6:243–250.

68 Calati R, Porcelli S, Giegling I, Hartmann AM, Möller HJ, De Ronchi D, Serretti A, Rujescu D: Catechol-O-methyltransferase gene modulation on suicidal behavior and personality traits: review, meta-analysis and association study. J Psychiatr Res 2011;45:309–321.

69 Tovilla-Zárate C, Juárez-Rojop I, Ramón-Frias T, Villar-Soto M, Pool-García S, Medellín BC, Genis Mendoza AD, Narvaez LL, Humberto N: No association between COMT val158met polymorphism and suicidal behavior: meta-analysis and new data. BMC Psychiatry 2011;11:151.

70 Zai CC, Manchia M, De Luca V, Tiwari AK, Chowdhury NI, Zai GC, Tong RP, Yilmaz Z, Shaikh SA, Strauss J, Kennedy JL: The brain-derived neurotrophic factor gene in suicidal behaviour: a meta-analysis. Int J Neuropsychopharmacol 2012;15:1037–1042.

71 Laje G, Allen AS, Akula N, Manji H, John Rush A, McMahon FJ: Genome-wide association study of suicidal ideation emerging during citalopram treatment of depressed outpatients. Pharmacogenet Genomics 2009;19:666–674.

72 Perroud N, Uher R, Ng MY, Guipponi M, Hauser J, Henigsberg N, Maier W, Mors O, Gennarelli M, Rietschel M, Souery D, Dernovsek MZ, Stamp AS, Lathrop M, Farmer A, Breen G, Aitchison KJ, Lewis CM, Craig IW, McGuffin P: Genome-wide association study of increasing suicidal ideation during antidepressant treatment in the GENDEP project. Pharmacogenomics J 2012;12:68–77.

73 Menke A, Domschke K, Czamara D, Klengel T, Hennings J, Lucae S, Baune BT, Arolt V, Müller-Myhsok B, Holsboer F, Binder EB: Genome-wide association study of antidepressant treatment-emergent suicidal ideation. Neuropsychopharmacology 2012;37:797–807.

74 Perlis RH, Huang J, Purcell S, Fava M, Rush AJ, Sullivan PF, Hamilton SP, McMahon FJ, Schulze TG, Potash JB, Zandi PP, Willour VL, Penninx BW, Boomsma DI, Vogelzangs N, Middeldorp CM, Rietschel M, Nöthen M, Cichon S, Gurling H, Bass N, McQuillin A, Hamshere M; Wellcome Trust Case Control Consortium Bipolar Disorder Group, Craddock N, Sklar P, Smoller JW: Genome-wide association study of suicide attempts in mood disorder patients. Am J Psychiatry 2010;167:1499–1507.

75 Schosser A, Butler AW, Ising M, Perroud N, Uher R, Ng MY, Cohen-Woods S, Craddock N, Owen MJ, Korszun A, Jones L, Jones I, Gill M, Rice JP, Maier W, Mors O, Rietschel M, Lucae S, Binder EB, Preisig M, Perry J, Tozzi F, Muglia P, Aitchison KJ, Breen G, Craig IW, Farmer AE, Müller-Myhsok B, McGuffin P, Lewis CM: Genome-wide association scan of suicidal thoughts and behaviour in major depression. PLoS One 2011;6:e20690.

76 Willour VL, Seifuddin F, Mahon PB, Jancic D, Pirooznia M, Steele J, Schweizer B, Goes FS, Mondimore FM, Mackinnon DF; Bipolar Genome Study Consortium, Perlis RH, Lee PH, Huang J, Kelsoe JR, Shilling PD, Rietschel M, Nöthen M, Cichon S, Gurling H, Purcell S, Smoller JW, Craddock N, DePaulo JR Jr, Schulze TG, McMahon FJ, Zandi PP, Potash JB: A genome-wide association study of attempted suicide. Mol Psychiatry 2012;17:433–444.

77 Mullins N, Perroud N, Uher R, Butler AW, Cohen-Woods S, Rivera M, Malki K, Euesden J, Power RA, Tansey KE, Jones L, Jones I, Craddock N, Owen MJ, Korszun A, Gill M, Mors O, Preisig M, Maier W, Rietschel M, Rice JP, Müller-Myhsok B, Binder EB, Lucae S, Ising M, Craig IW, Farmer AE, McGuffin P, Breen G, Lewis CM: Genetic relationships between suicide attempts, suicidal ideation and major psychiatric disorders: a genome-wide association and polygenic scoring study. Am J Med Genet B Neuropsychiatr Genet 2014;165B:428–437.

78 Zai CC, Gonçalves VF, Tiwari AK, Gagliano SA, Hosang G, de Luca V, Shaikh SA, King N, Chen Q, Xu W, Strauss J, Breen G, Lewis CM, Farmer AE, McGuffin P, Knight J, Vincent JB, Kennedy JL: A genome-wide association study of suicide severity scores in bipolar disorder. J Psychiatr Res 2015;65:23–29.

79 Galfalvy H, Haghighi F, Hodgkinson C, Goldman D, Oquendo MA, Burke A, Huang YY, Giegling I, Rujescu D, Bureau A, Turecki G, Mann JJ: A genome-wide association study of suicidal behavior. Am J Med Genet B Neuropsychiatr Genet 2015, Epub ahead of print.

Dan Rujescu
Department of Psychiatry, Psychotherapy and Psychosomatics
Martin Luther University Halle-Wittenberg
Julius-Kühn-Strasse 7
DE–06112 Halle (Germany)
E-Mail dan.rujescu@uk-halle.de

Kaschka WP, Rujescu D (eds): Biological Aspects of Suicidal Behavior.
Adv Biol Psychiatry. Basel, Karger, 2016, vol 30, pp 63–74 (DOI: 10.1159/000434737)

Gene-Environment Interaction Studies in Suicidal Behaviour

Laura Mandelli · Alessandro Serretti

Psychiatry Section, Department of Biomedical and Neuromotor Sciences, University of Bologna, Bologna, Italy

Abstract

Increasing evidence supports the involvement of both heritable and environmental risk factors in suicidal behaviour (SB). Gene-environment interaction (G × E) studies may be useful for elucidating the role of biological mechanisms in the risk for mental disorders. In the present article, we will review the literature regarding the interaction between genes modulating brain functions and stressful life events in the aetiology of SB (G × E studies) and discuss their potential added benefit compared to genetic studies only. Within the context of G × E investigation thus far, only a few reliable results have been obtained. However, since traditional G × E studies overall suffer from important methodological limitations, further effort is required to develop novel methodological strategies with an interdisciplinary approach.

Suicidal behaviour (SB) is an important public health issue, not only because of its often devastating consequences for the suicidal subject and his/her loved ones, but also because of its high prevalence and incidence in the population [1]. According to the World Health Organization [2], over 800,000 people die due to suicide every year and there are many more who attempt suicide. Suicide occurs throughout the lifespan and was the second leading cause of death globally in 2012 among those aged 15–29 years. The annual global age-standardized suicide rate is 11.4 per 100,000 population (15.0 for males and 8.0 for females). Social, psychological, cultural, and other factors can interact to lead a person to suicidal acts. Although SB can occur in different psychopathological conditions, patients affected by major depressive disorders (MDD) have the highest risk of attempting or committing suicide [3]. However, though extensive literature exists documenting an important overlap between MDD and SB with regard to familial risk, treatment and environmental risk factors, it has also been reported that SB may aggregate in families independently from the familial transmission of MDD [4], suggesting that independent genetic risk factors for SB may exist. The heritability and the estimated risk factors in relatives for SB is less clear than that of other mental disorders, also because SB mostly occurs within the context of other psychopathological conditions. However, twin studies have consistently documented genetic influences in SB, even when accounting for the effects of psychopathology. Concordance rates ranging from 6 to 35% have been reported in different studies of identical twins [5]. A number of biological factors and candidate genes have been tested in SB [6–9]. However, to date, only few consistent findings have been reported. One major challenge is that SB is a complex behaviour that may be produced by a combination of variations in multiple genes together with environmental factors, which modulate or trigger an existing genetic predisposition [10, 11]. For this reason, in the early 2000s, researchers have focused on studying the interplay between genetics and environmental risk factors. Gene-environment interaction (G × E) studies are useful in identifying interactive effects between genetic risk and environmental factors [12]. In addition to providing a better characterization of candidate genes, these studies may enable the identification of genes, which effects are dependent on the level of exposure to a specific environment. In the present chapter, after a brief review of the genetic factors involved in SB, we will review the studies focused on G × E in SB, highlighting the major and interesting findings obtained thus far. For this purpose, published G × E studies in SB were screened using several literature search strategies. Up to December 2014, appropriate search terms (gene, genetics, heritability, suicide, suicide attempt, completed suicide, suicidality, suicidal behaviour, suicidal ideation, and suicide intent) were entered into the common scientific literature databases (PubMed, Scopus and ISI Web of Science). The same terms were also entered in conjunction with other terms for G × E studies (stress, trauma, life events, adverse events, sexual abuse, physical abuse, emotional abuse, emotional neglect, and physical neglect). The reference lists of all the retrieved studies were reviewed in order to retrieve further relevant studies. The literature search was limited to reports in the English language.

Genetic Basis of Suicidal Behaviour

A number of candidate genes in SB have been tested in several studies, most frequently examining candidates related to the risk for MDD and involved in monoamine signalling, immunology/inflammation processes, neurotrophins, and neuroendocrinological factors. Genes that have been more or less consistently associated with SB (found positive in 2 or more independent studies and/or reported as associated in large meta-analyses) are reported in table 1.

Several genes such as serotonin transporter (SLC6A4), serotonin receptor 2A (5HTR2A), neuronal tryptophan hydroxylase (TPH2), brain-derived neurotrophic

Table 1. Genes associated with the risk for MDD and SB

Biological system/process	Gene	SB
Serotonin	SLC6A4	+
Serotonin	HTR2A	±
Serotonin	TPH2	+
Dopamine	DRD2	+
Noradrenalin	ADRA2A	+
Dopamine/noradrenalin	COMT	±
CNS prosurvival factor	BDNF	+
Lipid transporter	APOE	±
Blood pressure regulation	ACE	+

The genes, except for DRD2 and ADRA2A, have also been consistently associated with MDD. SB: + indicates consistent association; ± indicates uncertain association.

factor (BDNF), and others have also been reported as risk genes for MDD. This is not surprising since the majority of genetic studies in SB were performed on suicide attempters/completers suffering from depressive disorders compared to healthy (control) individuals. Nevertheless, studies comparing patients with SB to patients without SB (all affected by some psychopathology) have been performed as well, and some genes have been found positive in SB but not in MDD [13].

Gene Environment Interaction Studies in Suicidal Behaviour

Main Monoaminergic Central Systems (Serotonin, Dopamine and Noradrenalin)

A common polymorphism within SLC6A4 (5HTTLPR) has been the focus of much investigation in psychiatric disorders, especially in MDD and SB. Thus, it is not surprising that the pioneering G × E study in MDD by Caspi et al. [14] investigated this polymorphism. The study provided evidence that the short variant increased depressive symptoms, the risk of developing a depressive episode and also suicidal ideation after exposure to stressful life events (SLEs) in a large prospective community cohort. Subsequently, several studies have attempted to replicate this finding on depressive symptoms, MDD and correlated traits, with different measures of environmental risk for depression, and mixed results were obtained. Focussing on SB, studies confirmed the original finding of Caspi et al. of increased suicidal ideation after exposure to 2 or more SLEs in 5HTTLPR short-allele carriers. In particular, significant effects were observed in samples exposed to childhood maltreatment [15], childhood trauma [16], child abuse and severe SLEs [17, 18], school-aged children exposed to maltreatment [19], and community seniors [20]. However, Zalsman et al. [21], though confirming the interactive effect on depressive risk, failed to find the same effect on suicidal ideation. In community samples, Coventry et al. [22] failed to detect interactive effects on both MDD and SB. Nevertheless, a recent study confirmed an interaction between 5HTTLPR and childhood abuse on the risk for SB in a sample of MDD patients and found that the opposite variant (the long-long genotype) confers a higher risk for SB in individuals exposed to childhood abuse. Despite these inconsistencies, 6 out of 9 studies indicated that the 5HTTLPR genotype moderates the effect of stress on SB risk. However, with the exception of the first report by Caspi et al. [14] in 2003, 6 positive studies investigated psychiatric samples and 2 negative studies were performed on community samples. Thus, one may hypothesize that the interactive effect on SB is specific in the context of a pre-existing mental disorder. Conversely, we may also postulate that as suicide rates are lower in community samples compared to those in psychiatric samples, the power to detect true significant effects is decreased and true positives may have been missed. Other interesting genes investigated in G × E studies in both MDD and SB are 5HTR1A and 5HTR2A. Almost all studies focusing on 5HTR1A focused on the promoter polymorphism rs6295(C>G); 2 out of 4 studies reported interactive effects in SB, although these positive studies reported different alleles of risk (G allele in suicide attempters [23] and the CC genotype in suicide completers [24]). Therefore, clear conclusions regarding the potential role of this polymorphism in modulating the effect of environmental risk in SB cannot be drawn. A second polymorphism of interest in 5HTR1A is rs878567T>C. The minor C allele has been reported to have no direct effects on SB but may exhibit environmentally mediated effects [13]. Unfortunately, only 1 study, to our knowledge, took into account this variant in a G × E investigation. In the case of positive replication, this genetic variant would be of interest for predicting SB in individuals exposed to traumas early in life. G × E investigations on 5HTR2A produced conflicting results as well: two variants of the promoter polymorphism rs6313 (102T>C) provided some evidence of interactive effects in SB [25], although not consistently [24]. The rs7997012 was also found to interact with child abuse on SB in MDD patients [26]. Brezo et al. [13] reported three variants (rs7997012, rs6561333 and rs1885884) interacting with early trauma in SB but not in MDD. It is likely that such inconsistencies could be due to varied measures of environmental risk. However, because of the low number of studies performed, further studies are required to elucidate the role of this gene in modulating environmental risk and to identify the type of environmental risk in SB. Other genes encoding for serotoninergic receptors were poorly investigated in the G × E study, with mainly negative results. The tryptophan-hydroxylase genes TPH1 and TPH2 represent excellent candidates for investigation in G × E studies in SB, since they have been associated with this phenotype, particularly TPH2. Nevertheless, to our knowledge, only 2 G × E investigations have been published taking into account different genetic variations in TPH1 combined with childhood trauma [13, 24] but no positive interactive effects were detected. Similarly, neuronal TPH2 demonstrated poor evidence of interactive effects with environmental risk factors in MDD and SB – out of 3 studies, only 1 found an interaction between the rs7305115A>G variant and recent SLEs in SB risk in MDD patients [27]. Interestingly, in this study, the A allele in rs7305115 demonstrated a protective effect against SB in MDD patients exposed to recent SLEs. In view of the paucity of positive findings obtained, particularly with regard to TPH2, the potential environmental modulation of TPH2 and TPH1 deserves much more exploration. The dopaminergic and noradrenergic systems have also been investigated in the pathophysiology of depressive disorders and SB [28]. In particular, the dopamine receptor D2 (DRD2) has been consistently implicated in SB, while less evidence has been reported for MDD. However, to the best of our knowledge, no G × E study focusing on DRD2 in SB has been performed. In 1 study only, a positive interaction between the dopamine transporter (SLC6A3) and perceived maternal rejection in adolescents was found in SB risk [29]. Nevertheless, considering a different genetic variant within SLC6A3, another study found no evidence of an interactive effect with early sexual/physical abuse in adults [24]. Therefore, different environmental risks should be further investigated in association with SLC6A3 and SB. Regarding the noradrenergic system, only two genes have been investigated in a G × E study [24] – the noradrenalin transporter (SLC6A2) and the dopamine β-hydroxylase (DBH), which catalyzes the oxidative hydroxylation of dopamine to noradrenalin. However, no interactive effects with experience of sexual/physical abuse in childhood were detected on SB. Two genes involved in the metabolism (degradation) of monoamines have been consistently involved in MDD as well as other mental diseases in classical association studies – monoamine oxidase A (MAOA), which is involved in the metabolism of serotonin and noradrenalin, and catechol-O-methyltransferase (COMT), which is involved in the metabolism of dopamine and noradrenalin. Within the context of G × E studies, 3 published studies focused on SB and MAOA; all reported no interactive effects. This is consistent with simple association studies, which found that MAOA consistently involved in depressive disorders but not in SB. Similarly, no evidence has been reported for COMT in G × E studies in SB [24]. Nevertheless, Perroud et al. [30], by studying a sample of suicide attempters, found increased levels of anger in carriers of the Val allele in the rs4680 polymorphism (158Val>Met, considered as a protective variant against MDD), but only in individuals exposed to abuse in childhood. This finding may indicate that the protective variant for MDD may increase SB-related phenotypes (aggressiveness) in combination with early adversity.

Glutamatergic and GABAergic Endocannabinoid Genes

Genes involved in these systems have been investigated to a lower extent in MDD and SB in traditional genomic studies. However, the role of glutamate in modulating various mood states has been increasingly recognized [31]. Similarly, the GABA hypothesis of depression has found increasing support [32]. Further, the endocannabinoid system is known to participate in the control of emotional behaviour and mood [33]. In the context of G × E, only a few studies, to our knowledge, have investigated genes related to these systems in SB; 2 recent studies investigated some variants within genes pertaining to glutamate and GABA systems in combination with exposure to early adversity as potentially modulating the risk for SB, but no significant effects were observed [24, 34], although a combination of linked alleles in glutamate receptor 2B (GRIN2B) was found more frequently in suicide attempters compared to non-suicide attempters, independent of early adversity [34]. In addition, 1 study only focused on cannabinoid receptor 1 (CNUMBER1) in combination with environmental risk in SB but it failed to identify interactive effects in SB [24]. However, further studies are required to elucidate the role of this gene in SB and in combination with environmental adverse exposure.

Corticotrophin-Related Genes

Hyperdrive of corticotrophin-releasing hormone (CRH) has long been considered a fundamental neurobiological correlate of MDD [35]. However, thus far, genomic studies have found little evidence for this factor in MDD, particularly with regard to the major candidate gene encoding for CRH receptor 1 (CRHR1). Nevertheless, some evidence has supported the significant role of this gene within the context of G × E studies, although highly mixed results were obtained [19, 36–40]. Mixed results were also obtained in the context of SB, where the genetic variants investigated were found not to interact with environmental stress in some studies [24, 41], to increase SB risk in low-stressed individuals [42] or to decrease it in early traumatized individuals [43]. Given these results, albeit conflicting, the CRHR1 may be reliably implicated in the modulation of environmental effects on mental and behavioural psychopathology but it is likely that a complex combination of mutations, timing of SLEs and interactions with other genetic effects (epistasis) have to be considered in further studies. Furthermore, two G × E studies investigated genetic variants in other genes involved in the central corticotrophin system such as the gene encoding for CRH [41, 42], CRH receptor 2 (CRHR2) and CRH-binding protein (CRHBP). However, little evidence has been obtained, with the exception of CRHBP. Indeed, a variant in CRHBP was found to increase the risk for SB in combination with childhood trauma [41]. However, further studies are required to confirm this finding.

Genes Involved in Neurotrophic Processes

Genes encoding for prosurvival factors in CNS cells, neurotrophins and proteins promoting cellular survival and proliferation are thought to be important mediators of cellular alterations observed in psychiatric disorders and mental/behavioural disturbances [44]. In recent years, a large number of studies have focused on BDNF, with consistent evidence of its involvement in both MDD and SB. This gene, together with the 5-HTTLPR polymorphism in SLC6A4, was also the most investigated gene in G × E studies. Evidence has been reported that the Met or G allele in the rs6265 polymorphism of BDNF may be a risk factor for MDD in combination with exposure to environmental adversity [45–57]. Conversely, the 'protective' Val (or A allele) has been associated with an increased risk for SB in combination with exposure to environmental stress [58–60]. As previously discussed, similar opposite effects of alleles in MDD and SB were reported for the rs4680 (158Val>Met) variant in the COMT gene. These findings may suggest that genetic variations within BDNF also differentially affect intermediate phenotypes, eliciting individuals to exhibit different pathological responses to stress. However, it is not easy to draw clear hypotheses. BDNF binds to the tyrosine kinase receptor B (NTRK2). Genetic variations for NTRK2 have been implicated in both MDD [61] and SB [62]. Recently, Murphy et al. [24] found a common genotype (C/C) in NTRK2 to increase the risk for SB in individuals exposed to early trauma. However, we found no other studies in the literature supporting or contrasting this result. Ornithine decarboxylase (ODC) is the first committed step in the synthesis of polyamines, which are important factors for stabilizing DNA structures and for the DNA double-strand break repair pathway and which function as antioxidants [63]. A recent study by Sokolowski et al. [34] found a variant in ODC1 (rs7559979) to increase the risk of severe suicide attempts in individuals exposed to physical assault in childhood/adolescence. This finding is of interest, since it indicates that a new gene that has never been investigated in MDD may be relevant for SB.

Genes Involved in Inflammatory Processes

There is evidence that MDD is associated with inflammation and cell-mediated immune activation [64]. However, the majority of simple genetic association studies have not found relevant effects in MDD and SB and we were not able to detect G × E studies focussed on SB. Remarkably, the FK506-binding protein 5 gene (FKBP5), encoding for a protein belonging to immunophilins that may affect HPA axis functioning, has been shown to be involved in the recurrence of MDD, bipolar disorder, SB, and response to antidepressant treatment [65, 66]. Two studies by Roy et al. [41, 67] reported that genetic variations within FKBP5 interact with early adversity in increasing the risk for SB, particularly with regard to the 3′-UTR rs3800373(G>T) polymorphism.

Other Genes

Some evidence has been reported for regulators of G-protein signalling in SB and recent studies have suggested that the regulator of G-protein signalling 2 (RGS2) plays an important role in anxiety and/or aggressive behaviour. A post-mortem study indicated that genetic variations within RGS2 are potentially involved in the susceptibility to SB [68]. According to Amstadter et al. [69], the rs4606 variant, reported by Cui et al. [68] to be associated with complete suicide, was more common in individuals who developed suicidal ideation after exposure to hurricanes in Florida in 2004. This preliminary evidence may indicate that RGS2 is involved in SB after exposure to severe adverse life events. Finally, G × E studies have investigated other genes in SB, including the arginine vasopressin receptor 1B (AVPR1B), which is involved in the release of acetylcholine, prolactin and endorphins [70], and the ATP-binding cassette, subfamily G, member 1 (ABCG1), which encodes for an ATP-binding cassette transporter involved in multi-drug resistance, but did not indicate any evidence of interactive effects with environmental risk [24].

Discussion and Conclusions

It has been well recognized that single genes may not explain the full risk of developing complex diseases and that heritable factors, when taken together, may account for approximately 50% of the variance in risk [71]. Evolutionary forces rapidly eliminate large gene effects and complex highly prevalent diseases are associated with minor gene effects [72]. Thus, it is more likely that genes with small interacting genetic effects, in conjunction with environmental factors, affect the risk for complex disorders such as psychiatric diseases [73]. Far from being the best model to investigate the pathogenesis of mental disease, G × E studies have long advocated for combining biological factors and environmental risk [74]. In this chapter, our focus was specifically on G × E studies in SB. The effect of some genes on SB risk appears to be to some extent influenced by the exposure to environmental risk, particularly with regard to 5HTTLPR, BDNF, CRH, SLC6A2, and COMT, though with mixed evidence. Despite the preliminary nature of these studies and the inability to reliably disentangle specific interactive effects in SB, useful and additional information can be obtained from these studies. G × E studies may allow the discovery of a causal role for genes that contribute only slightly to a specific disorder that can change in effect size depending on the individual exposure to environmental risk or other individual characteristics. Furthermore, G × E studies may provide additional evidence for genes that have already been consistently associated with specific mental disorders and may provide evidence for a gene's causal role, resulting in different abnormal phenotypes in individuals, depending on the type of risk environment that they have been exposed to or the timing in life of the exposure. An additional advantage of G × E studies, when studying correlated mental/behaviour disturbance, is the possibility of observing the risk-increasing effect for one phenotype and the protective effect for another phenotype in the same variant. Finally, G × E investigations may also confirm direct effects found in simple genetic association studies (not mediated by environmental exposure).

In summary, although the G × E approach is far from being the leading methodology used to investigate biological and psychosocial risk factors in psychiatric diseases, the approach has a number of advantages that have motivated several biological researchers since the early 2000s to investigate the interplay between genes and environmental risk factors. However, this field of investigation is rather new and few quality studies have been conducted thus far, especially in the context of SB. This type of investigation suffers from a number of methodological limitations such as the high number of potential statistical tests required to examine interaction effects, the high likelihood of obtaining random positive effects because of the multiple possibilities for grouping genotypes and testing different polymorphisms, heterogeneity between studies due to the sampling of different populations across which the genetic effects of interest may vary in strength or direction, heterogeneity in the investigated phenotype and environment, or heterogeneity in the measure of the same phenotype/environment due to the employment of a different tool of evaluation [75–78]. Thus, more complex and reliable methods of investigation should be developed in order to overcome such limitations in G × E studies.

References

1 Borges G, Nock MK, Haro Abad JM, et al: Twelve-month prevalence of and risk factors for suicide attempts in the World Health Organization World Mental Health Surveys. J Clin Psychiatry 2010;71:1617–1628.
2 World Health Organization: Preventing Suicide: A Global Imperative. Luxemburg, WHO, 2014.
3 Harrison PJ, Burnet PW: The 5-HT2A (serotonin2A) receptor gene in the aetiology, pathophysiology and pharmacotherapy of schizophrenia. J Psychopharmacol 1997;11:18–20.
4 Brent DA, Mann JJ: Familial pathways to suicidal behavior – understanding and preventing suicide among adolescents. New Engl J Med 2006;355:2719–2721.
5 Pedersen NL, Fiske A: Genetic influences on suicide and nonfatal suicidal behavior: twin study findings. Eur Psychiatry 2010;25:264–267.
6 Antypa N, Serretti A, Rujescu D: Serotonergic genes and suicide: a systematic review. Eur Neuropsychopharmacol 2013;23:1125–1142.
7 Boulougouris V, Malogiannis I, Lockwood G, et al: Serotonergic modulation of suicidal behaviour: integrating preclinical data with clinical practice and psychotherapy. Exp Brain Res 2013;230:605–624.
8 Rujescu D, Thalmeier A, Moeller H-J, et al: Molecular genetic findings in suicidal behavior; what is beyond the serotonergic system? Arch Suicide Res 2007;11:17–40.
9 Tsai SJ, Hong CJ, Liou YJ: Recent molecular genetic studies and methodological issues in suicide research. Prog Neuropsychopharmacol Biol Psychiatry 2011;35:809–817.
10 Roy A, Sarchiopone M, Carli V: Gene-environment interaction and suicidal behavior. J Psychiatr Pract 2009;15:282–288.
11 Saveanu RV, Nemeroff CB: Etiology of depression: genetic and environmental factors. Psychiatr Clin North Am 2012;35:51–71.
12 Cooper B: Nature, nurture and mental disorder: old concepts in the new millennium. Br J Psychiatry 2001;40:s91–s101.
13 Brezo J, Bureau A, Merette C, et al: Differences and similarities in the serotonergic diathesis for suicide attempts and mood disorders: a 22-year longitudinal gene-environment study. Mol Psychiatry 2010;15:831–843.
14 Caspi A, Sugden K, Moffitt TE, et al: Influence of life stress on depression: moderation by a polymorphism in the 5-HTT gene. Science 2003;301:386–389.
15 Gibb BE, McGeary JE, Beevers CG, et al: Serotonin transporter (5-HTTLPR) genotype, childhood abuse, and suicide attempts in adult psychiatric inpatients. Suicide Life Threat Behav 2006;36:687–693.
16 Roy A, Hu XZ, Janal MN, et al: Interaction between childhood trauma and serotonin transporter gene variation in suicide. Neuropsychopharmacology 2007;32:2046–2052.
17 Peyrot WJ, Middeldorp CM, Jansen R, et al: Strong effects of environmental factors on prevalence and course of major depressive disorder are not moderated by 5-HTTLPR polymorphisms in a large Dutch sample. J Affect Disord 2013;146:91–99.
18 Shinozaki G, Romanowicz M, Passov V, et al: State dependent gene-environment interaction: serotonin transporter gene-child abuse interaction associated with suicide attempt history among depressed psychiatric inpatients. J Affect Disord 2013;147:373–378.
19 Cicchetti D, Rogosch FA, Sturge-Apple ML: Interactions of child maltreatment and serotonin transporter and monoamine oxidase A polymorphisms: depressive symptomatology among adolescents from low socioeconomic status backgrounds. Dev Psychopathol 2007;19:1161–1180.
20 Kim JM, Stewart R, Kim SW, et al: Interactions between a serotonin transporter gene, life events and social support on suicidal ideation in Korean elders. J Affect Disord 2014;160:14–20.

21 Zalsman G, Huang YY, Oquendo MA, et al: Association of a triallelic serotonin transporter gene promoter region (5-HTTLPR) polymorphism with stressful life events and severity of depression. Am J Psychiatry 2006;163:1588–1593.
22 Coventry WL, James MR, Eaves LJ, et al: Do 5HTTLPR and stress interact in risk for depression and suicidality? Item response analyses of a large sample. Am J Med Genet B Neuropsychiatr Genet 2010;153B:757–765.
23 Wasserman D, Geijer T, Sokolowski M, et al: The serotonin 1A receptor C(-1019)G polymorphism in relation to suicide attempt. Behav Brain Funct 2006; 2:14.
24 Murphy TM, Ryan M, Foster T, et al: Risk and protective genetic variants in suicidal behaviour: association with SLC1A2, SLC1A3, 5-HTR1B and NTRK2 polymorphisms. Behav Brain Funct 2011;7: 22.
25 Ben-Efraim YJ, Wasserman D, Wasserman J, et al: Family-based study of HTR2A in suicide attempts: observed gene, gene × environment and parent-of-origin associations. Mol Psychiatry 2013;18:758–766.
26 Shinozaki G, Romanowicz M, Mrazek DA, et al: HTR2A gene-child abuse interaction and association with a history of suicide attempt among Caucasian depressed psychiatric inpatients. J Affect Disord 2013;150:1200–1203.
27 Zhang Y, Zhang C, Yuan G, et al: Effect of tryptophan hydroxylase-2 rs7305115 SNP on suicide attempts risk in major depression. Behav Brain Funct 2010;6:49.
28 El Mansari M, Guiard BP, Chernoloz O, et al: Relevance of norepinephrine-dopamine interactions in the treatment of major depressive disorder. CNS Neurosci Ther 2010;16:e1–e17.
29 Haeffel GJ, Getchell M, Koposov RA, et al: Association between polymorphisms in the dopamine transporter gene and depression: evidence for a gene-environment interaction in a sample of juvenile detainees. Psychol Sci 2008;19:62–69.
30 Perroud N, Jaussent I, Guillaume S, et al: COMT but not serotonin-related genes modulates the influence of childhood abuse on anger traits. Genes Brain Behav 2010;9:193–202.
31 Owen RT: Glutamatergic approaches in major depressive disorder: focus on ketamine, memantine and riluzole. Drugs Today (Barc) 2012;48:469–478.
32 Mohler H: The GABA system in anxiety and depression and its therapeutic potential. Neuropharmacology 2012;62:42–53.
33 Esteban S, Garcia-Sevilla JA: Effects induced by cannabinoids on monoaminergic systems in the brain and their implications for psychiatric disorders. Progr Neuropsychopharmacol Biol Psychiatry 2012; 38:78–87.
34 Sokolowski M, Ben-Efraim YJ, Wasserman J, et al: Glutamatergic GRIN2B and polyaminergic ODC1 genes in suicide attempts: associations and gene-environment interactions with childhood/adolescent physical assault. Mol Psychiatry 2013;18:985–992.
35 Claes SJ: CRH, stress, and major depression: a psychobiological interplay. Vitam Horm 2004;69:117–150.
36 Bradley RG, Binder EB, Epstein MP, et al: Influence of child abuse on adult depression: moderation by the corticotropin-releasing hormone receptor gene. Arch Gen Psychiatry 2008;65:190–200.
37 Grabe HJ, Schwahn C, Appel K, et al: Childhood maltreatment, the corticotropin-releasing hormone receptor gene and adult depression in the general population. Am J Med Genet B Neuropsychiatr Genet 2010;153B:1483–1493.
38 Heim C, Bradley B, Mletzko TC, et al: Effect of childhood trauma on adult depression and neuroendocrine function: sex-specific moderation by CRH receptor 1 gene. Front Behav Neurosci 2009;3:41.
39 Polanczyk G, Caspi A, Williams B, et al: Protective effect of CRHR1 gene variants on the development of adult depression following childhood maltreatment: replication and extension. Arch Gen Psychiatry 2009;66:978–985.
40 Ressler KJ, Bradley B, Mercer KB, et al: Polymorphisms in CRHR1 and the serotonin transporter loci: gene × gene × environment interactions on depressive symptoms. Am J Med Genet B Neuropsychiatr Genet 2010;153B:812–824.
41 Roy A, Hodgkinson CA, Deluca V, et al: Two HPA axis genes, CRHBP and FKBP5, interact with childhood trauma to increase the risk for suicidal behavior. J Psychiatr Res 2012;46:72–79.
42 Wasserman D, Sokolowski M, Rozanov V, et al: The CRHR1 gene: a marker for suicidality in depressed males exposed to low stress. Genes Brain Behav 2008; 7:14–19.
43 Ben-Efraim YJ, Wasserman D, Wasserman J, et al: Gene-environment interactions between CRHR1 variants and physical assault in suicide attempts. Genes Brain Behav 2011;10:663–672.
44 Castren E, Rantamaki T: Role of brain-derived neurotrophic factor in the aetiology of depression: implications for pharmacological treatment. CNS Drugs 2010;24:1–7.
45 Aguilera M, Arias B, Wichers M, et al: Early adversity and 5-HTT/BDNF genes: new evidence of gene-environment interactions on depressive symptoms in a general population. Psychol Med 2009;39:1425–1432.
46 Bukh JD, Bock C, Vinberg M, et al: Interaction between genetic polymorphisms and stressful life events in first episode depression. J Affect Disord 2009;119:107–115.

47 Chen J, Li X, McGue M: Interacting effect of BDNF Val66Met polymorphism and stressful life events on adolescent depression. Genes Brain Behav 2012;11: 958–965.
48 Gatt JM, Nemeroff CB, Schofield PR, et al: Early life stress combined with serotonin 3A receptor and brain-derived neurotrophic factor valine 66 to methionine genotypes impacts emotional brain and arousal correlates of risk for depression. Biol Psychiatry 2010;68:818–824.
49 Grabe HJ, Schwahn C, Mahler J, et al: Genetic epistasis between the brain-derived neurotrophic factor Val66Met polymorphism and the 5-HTT promoter polymorphism moderates the susceptibility to depressive disorders after childhood abuse. Progr Neuropsychopharmacol Biol Psychiatry 2012;36:264–270.
50 Hosang GM, Uher R, Keers R, et al: Stressful life events and the brain-derived neurotrophic factor gene in bipolar disorder. J Affect Disord 2010;125: 345–349.
51 Juhasz G, Dunham JS, McKie S, et al: The CREB1-BDNF-NTRK2 pathway in depression: multiple gene-cognition-environment interactions. Biol Psychiatry 2011;69:762–771.
52 Kaufman J, Yang BZ, Douglas-Palumberi H, et al: Brain-derived neurotrophic factor-5-HTTLPR gene interactions and environmental modifiers of depression in children. Biol Psychiatry 2006;59:673–680.
53 Lavebratt C, Aberg E, Sjoholm LK, et al: Variations in FKBP5 and BDNF genes are suggestively associated with depression in a Swedish population-based cohort. J Affect Disord 2010;125:249–255.
54 Perea CS, Paternina AC, Gomez Y, et al: Negative affectivity moderated by BDNF and stress response. J Affect Disord 2012;136:767–774.
55 Quinn CR, Dobson-Stone C, Outhred T, et al: The contribution of BDNF and 5-HTT polymorphisms and early life stress to the heterogeneity of major depressive disorder: a preliminary study. Aust NZ J Psychiatry 2012;46:55–63.
56 Wichers M, Kenis G, Jacobs N, et al: The BDNF Val(66)Met × 5-HTTLPR × child adversity interaction and depressive symptoms: an attempt at replication. Am J Med Genet B Neuropsychiatr Genet 2008; 147B:120–123.
57 Yang C, Xu Y, Sun N, et al.: The combined effects of the BDNF and GSK3B genes modulate the relationship between negative life events and major depressive disorder. Brain Res 2010;1355:1–6.
58 Bresin K, Sima Finy M, Verona E: Childhood emotional environment and self-injurious behaviors: the moderating role of the BDNF Val66Met polymorphism. J Affect Disord 2013;150:594–600.
59 Perroud N, Courtet P, Vincze I, et al: Interaction between BDNF Val66Met and childhood trauma on adult's violent suicide attempt. Genes Brain Behav 2008;7:314–322.
60 Sarchiapone M, Carli V, Roy A, et al: Association of polymorphism (Val66Met) of brain-derived neurotrophic factor with suicide attempts in depressed patients. Neuropsychobiology 2008;57:139–145.
61 Dong C, Wong ML, Licinio J: Sequence variations of ABCB1, SLC6A2, SLC6A3, SLC6A4, CREB1, CRHR1 and NTRK2: association with major depression and antidepressant response in Mexican-Americans. Mol Psychiatry 2009;14:1105–1118.
62 Perroud N, Aitchison KJ, Uher R, et al: Genetic predictors of increase in suicidal ideation during antidepressant treatment in the GENDEP project. Neuropsychopharmacology 2009;34:2517–2528.
63 Pendeville H, Carpino N, Marine JC, et al: The ornithine decarboxylase gene is essential for cell survival during early murine development. Mol Cell Biol 2001;21:6549–6558.
64 Leonard B, Maes M: Mechanistic explanations how cell-mediated immune activation, inflammation and oxidative and nitrosative stress pathways and their sequels and concomitants play a role in the pathophysiology of unipolar depression. Neurosci Biobehav Rev 2012;36:764–785.
65 Binder EB, Salyakina D, Lichtner P, et al: Polymorphisms in FKBP5 are associated with increased recurrence of depressive episodes and rapid response to antidepressant treatment. Nat Genet 2004;36: 1319–1325.
66 Willour VL, Chen H, Toolan J, et al: Family-based association of FKBP5 in bipolar disorder. Mol Psychiatry 2009;14:261–268.
67 Roy A, Gorodetsky E, Yuan Q, et al: Interaction of FKBP5, a stress-related gene, with childhood trauma increases the risk for attempting suicide. Neuropsychopharmacology 2010;35:1674–1683.
68 Cui H, Nishiguchi N, Ivleva E, et al: Association of RGS2 gene polymorphisms with suicide and increased RGS2 immunoreactivity in the postmortem brain of suicide victims. Neuropsychopharmacology 2008;33:1537–1544.
69 Amstadter AB, Koenen KC, Ruggiero KJ, et al: Variation in RGS2 is associated with suicidal ideation in an epidemiological study of adults exposed to the 2004 Florida hurricanes. Arch Suicide Res 2009;13: 349–357.
70 Ben-Efraim YJ, Wasserman D, Wasserman J, et al: Family-based study of AVPR1B association and interaction with stressful life events on depression and anxiety in suicide attempts. Neuropsychopharmacology 2013;38:1504–1511.
71 Kendler KS: Twin studies of psychiatric illness: an update. Arch Gen Psychiatry 2001;58:1005–1014.

72 Risch NJ: Mapping genes for psychiatric disorders; in Gershon ES, Cloninger CR (eds): Genetic Approaches to Mental Disorders. Washington, American Psychiatric Press, 1994.

73 Sanders AR, Duan J, Gejman PV: Complexities in psychiatric genetics. Int Rev Psychiatry 2004;16:284–293.

74 Brock JF: Nature, nurture, and stress in health and disease. Lancet 1972;1:701–704.

75 Laucht M, Treutlein J, Blomeyer D, et al: Interaction between the 5-HTTLPR serotonin transporter polymorphism and environmental adversity for mood and anxiety psychopathology: evidence from a high-risk community sample of young adults. Int J Neuropsychopharmacol 2009;12:737–747.

76 Munafo MR, Durrant C, Lewis G, et al: Gene × environment interactions at the serotonin transporter locus. Biol Psychiatry 2009;65:211–219.

77 Munafo MR, Flint J: Replication and heterogeneity in gene × environment interaction studies. Int J Neuropsychopharmacol 2009;12:727–729.

78 Sullivan PF: Spurious genetic associations. Biol Psychiatry 2007;61:1121–1126.

Laura Mandelli, PhD
Psychiatry Section, Department of Biomedical and Neuromotor Sciences
University of Bologna
Viale C. Pepoli 5
IT–40123 Bologna (Italy)
E-Mail laura.mandelli@unibo.it

Kaschka WP, Rujescu D (eds): Biological Aspects of Suicidal Behavior.
Adv Biol Psychiatry. Basel, Karger, 2016, vol 30, pp 75–87 (DOI: 10.1159/000434738)

Epigenetics of Suicidal Behaviour

Gustavo Turecki

McGill Group for Suicide Studies, Douglas Mental Health University Institute, Department of Psychiatry, McGill University, Montreal, Que., Canada

Abstract

Epigenetics refers to the dynamic molecular processes that regulate gene expression by changing the chemical composition or physical structure of DNA or chromatin without altering its sequence. The aetiology of suicide is complex and there is substantial evidence supporting an association between early-life adversity and increased suicide risk. Indeed, the early-life environment has important consequences on behavioural development and only recently have we started to uncover some of the mechanisms accounting for the behavioural changes induced by early-life adversity. The epigenome is responsive to the environment and thus, through epigenetic regulation, early-life adversity is capable of altering behavioural development and increasing the vulnerability toward psychopathology, including suicide. In this chapter we will review the findings in support of this view describing epigenetic changes associated with early-life adversity and suicide.

Suicide Risk and Early-Life Adversity

Although numerous models have been proposed over the years in attempting to understand suicide risk, most current models understand suicide as resulting from the interaction of several distal and proximal risk factors. At one end of the spectrum, risk factors acting more distally are those believed to increase predisposition while at the other end, risk factors acting more proximally are regarded as precipitants [1]. Examples of proximal factors are recent life events and the last 6-month psychopathology, including current substance abuse, while distal factors that are commonly studied include genetic make-up and early-life adversity. The latter is undoubtedly one of the distal factors with the most robust association with suicide risk [2–4].

Early-life experiences, including childhood abuse, can have a significant impact on an individual's susceptibility to suicide and suicidal behaviours. While most individuals who display suicidal behaviour do not have a history of early-life adversity, a significant minority of up to 40%, depending on the type of abuse, frequency and suicide phenotype, does [5–10]. Accordingly, several longitudinal studies conducted in epidemiologically representative samples consistently indicate that children who have histories of sexual and physical abuse during childhood are more likely to manifest suicidal behaviour in adulthood [2–4, 10–12]. Indeed, child trauma, and particularly child sexual and physical abuse, is associated with increased risk of psychiatric disorders, including depression, anxiety, bipolar disorder, substance abuse, and suicide [13–21].

While there is substantial evidence to support a link between early-life adversity and the development of psychopathology in adulthood, what long-lasting molecular changes occur as a result of adverse life experience that could increase the risk of suicide? In this chapter we will review the data suggesting that changes at the molecular level are occurring in response to variation in the early-life environment. Specifically, we focus on epigenetic processes as they are believed to regulate expression levels of genes that affect response systems and, in turn, modulate behaviour. Indeed, there is mounting evidence suggesting that epigenetic alterations in several key genes are occurring as a result of early-life adversity and these changes may be contributing to increased suicide risk. However, before proceeding any further we must first review some of the basic concepts of epigenetics.

Epigenetic Regulation of Gene Expression

Although the genome contains the entire genetic information required to express all the proteins of an entire organism, only a fraction of this information is expressed in a given cell at a given time. Epigenetics refers to the collective chemical and physical processes that program the genome to express its genes in a time- and cell-dependent manner. They are dynamic molecular processes that regulate gene expression by changing the chemical composition or physical structure of DNA or chromatin without altering its sequence. These also include modifications that affect the availability of mRNA products. The epigenome is responsive to developmental, physiological and environmental cues and in this way epigenetics provides a basis for understanding how the environment may regulate the genome. Epigenetic regulation of gene function allows for genomic plasticity, that is, the adaptation of the genome to the needs of the organism. It has long been clear that epigenetic processes occur as a result of physical and chemical environmental signals. However, only recently has it been revealed that the social environment also triggers epigenetic responses [22–24]. As such, it is possible to conceptualize the epigenome as an interface through which the environment can influence genetic processes and as a result regulate behaviour, at least partially, in response to environmental needs [1]. Among epigenetic mechanisms, the better characterized are DNA methylation, histone modifications and non-coding RNAs.

DNA Methylation

DNA methylation is the best characterized and most investigated among the variety of known epigenetic processes. DNA methylation is a posttranscriptional modification referring mainly to the transfer of a methyl group (CH_3) from an S-adenosyl-L-methionine donor to the 5′ carbon of the cytosine from dinucleotide sequences of cytosine-guanine (CpG), a process that requires the enzymatic activity of DNA methyltransferase (DNMT) proteins among which DNMT3a and DNMT3b are de novo methylases as they add methyl groups to cytosines that were not previously methylated [25, 26]. DNA methylation in the promoter region of a gene is associated with transcriptional repression of that gene by interference with the ability of transcription factors or similar proteins from binding to their target DNA regulatory sequences [27]. Another form of DNA methylation is DNA hydroxymethylation, which refers to the oxidation of pre-existing 5′-methylcytosine to 5′-hydroxymethylcytosine by enzymes in the TET family [28, 29]. Moreover, 5-hydroxymethylcytosine is an intermediate in DNA demethylation and its concentrations positively correlate with gene transcription [30].

Histone Modifications

DNA is compacted around an octamer of histone proteins (H2A, H2B, H3 and H4) that form nucleosomes, which constitute the fundamental units of chromatin. Histones are globular structures that have a tail of amino acids which can be modified by the addition or removal of chemical residues. Chromatin exists in two states: the active state, euchromatin, is associated with gene transcription and the inactive state, heterochromatin, corresponds to gene repression. The chromatin state is dynamically regulated by the recruitment of proteins carrying intrinsic enzymatic activity leading to histone modifications [31–35]. These modifications drive the chromatin opening or closing favouring an active or inactive state of chromatin [36, 37]. Histone acetyltransferases add acetyl groups to certain amino acid residues on histones while histone deacetylases catalyze the removal of acetyl groups [38]. Hyperacetylation of histone proteins leads to chromatin decondensation, which makes it looser and more accessible. Up to eight types of histone modifications have been characterized, as follows: methylation (lysine, arginine), acetylation, phosphorylation, ubiquitylation, sumoylation, deimination, ADP ribosylation, and proline isomerisation. While all these marks may affect gene expression, most of the focus has been on lysine methylation and acetylation. For instance, methylation at specific lysines (K) of the third histone (H), as in H3K4, H3K36 and H3K79, has been associated with active transcription [39–44], whereas methylation at H3K9, H3K27 and H4K20 has been reported to correlate with transcriptional repression [43, 45–51].

Non-Coding RNAs

There is mounting evidence that differential gene expression patterns may result from the action of non-coding RNAs that are capable of activating or repressing genes [52–54]. Among the different species of non-coding RNAs, microRNAs have been gaining significant interest as they are implicated in the posttranscriptional regulation of mRNA and, thus, can regulate gene expression. MicroRNAs are small, non-coding, single-stranded, 19- to 24-base RNA transcripts that bind to mRNAs and target them for degradation. RNA interference activity is a process in which microRNAs form complexes that target complementary mRNA leading to either translational repression or the degradation of the targeted transcript, which also results in gene repression [55].

The Hypothalamic-Pituitary-Adrenal Axis

Child abuse has been proposed to impose long-term effects on behaviour partly by altering the neural circuits involved in the regulation of stress [56]. The hypothalamic-pituitary-adrenal (HPA) axis is the main stress regulatory system [57]. There is evidence to suggest that early-life adversity is associated with structural and functional alterations to several brain regions implicated in the stress response [58–63]. Individuals with a history of child abuse exhibit altered stress responses [64, 65] and individuals exposed to childhood abuse, particularly physical abuse, exhibit increased corticotropin-releasing factor levels [56, 66]. In sum, there are several changes occurring in the HPA axis and these changes may be contributing to alterations in behaviour that may increase a predisposition to suicidal behaviour later in life.

The first evidence to suggest that the early-life environment induces changes in stable epigenetic states that regulate gene expression and, ultimately, complex neural functions was demonstrated in studies investigating the effect of variations in maternal care in rats on stress reactivity. In both rodents and non-human primates the early-life environment regulates HPA axis function in adulthood [67–70]. Landmark studies conducted by Meaney and colleagues [67, 68, 71, 72] demonstrated that variations in the early social environment, as modelled by maternal care in the rat (the frequency of pup licking/grooming, LG, over the first week of life), program the expression of genes that regulate behavioural and endocrine responses to stress. Specifically, these studies revealed that pups raised by mothers that exhibited increased frequency of pup LG (i.e. high-LG mothers) exhibited in adulthood increased hippocampal glucocorticoid receptor (GR; *NR3C1*) expression, greater negative feedback regulation over hypothalamic corticotropin-releasing factor and more modest responses to stress compared to the offspring of low-LG mothers [67, 71, 72]. Variations in maternal LG were found to be linked to an epigenetic modification of a neuron-specific exon 1_7 promoter of GR [67] such that increased maternal care is associated with decreased methylation of the $GR1_7$ promoter and increased hippocampal GR expression. This research underlines the profound and persistent impact that differential early-life experiences can have on gene expression and behaviour through epigenetic mechanisms and DNA methylation changes, thus providing strong support for the ability of the early environment to stably influence neurodevelopment and complex behavioural traits.

Subsequent work has provided evidence that the GR methylation findings reported in rats translate to humans. These changes contribute to the emergence into adulthood of maladaptive stress responses and potentiate the risk of suicide. Accordingly, the first evidence for an effect of early-life adversity on the epigenetic state of the human genome was observed investigating the methylation state of the GR gene in the hippocampus of individuals who died by suicide and had histories of child abuse. In particular, early-life adversity in humans reprograms the DNA methylation patterns of one particular GR gene transcript variant, the $GR1_F$ ($GR1_7$ homologue in rats) promoter. Increased methylation in the $GR1_F$ promoter region and decreased $GR1_F$ expression was found in the hippocampus of suicide completers with a history of child abuse compared to non-abused suicide completers and healthy controls [73]. This hypermethylation reduced NGFI-A transcription factor binding, probably accounting for decreased GR expression. Given that decreased GR expression is known to result in HPA axis hyperactivity, there is strong evidence implicating the role of childhood abuse in the disruption of this key stress response system. As such, the evidence highly implicates HPA axis dysregulation in the aetiology of suicide following a history of severe early-life adversity.

This investigation was later extended to other transcripts of GR. The GR gene is preceded by non-coding exons and in humans 9 first-exon variants each possessing their own promoter region have been identified, as follows: $1_{A, I, D, J, E, B, F, C \text{ and } H}$ [74]. Expression of the non-coding exons 1_B, 1_C and 1_H was found to be significantly decreased in the hippocampus of suicide completers with a history of childhood abuse compared to non-abused suicide completers and controls [75]. This assessment revealed that $GR1_C$ promoter methylation levels are inversely correlated with $GR1_C$ expression in accordance with the previous finding on the 1_F variant, whereas the $GR1_H$ promoter showed site-specific hypomethylation that was positively correlated with $GR1_H$ expression. This suggests that active demethylation is also a functional mechanism that could be affected by early-life adversity. While this is a mechanism that has received less attention, more work is required in order to elucidate its potential implications in the context of early-life adversity.

These findings have been supported by several groups investigating peripheral blood samples from different populations of individuals who were exposed to varying forms of early-life adversity. Infants of mothers who reported suffering intimate partner violence during pregnancy exhibited higher levels of methylation in the promoter of $GR1_F$ compared to those born from mothers without such treatment [76]. In another study significant correlations were found between $GR1_F$ promoter methylation levels and parental loss, child maltreatment and parental care such that diminished nurturing was associated with increased methylation of this gene [77]. In addition, another group reported that childhood maltreatment, its severity and the type of abuse and frequency were positively correlated with $GR1_F$ promoter methylation levels [78, 79]. Altogether, the evidence seems to suggest that early-life adversity is capable of inducing specific long-lasting epigenetic alterations that ultimately affect gene expression.

In a different study assessing the expression of several GR exon 1 variants expressed in the limbic tissue of depressed suicide completers, $GR1_F$ and $GR1_C$ hippocampal expression was significantly decreased without any report of promoter hypermethylation [80]. However, the investigation was carried out only in a limited region of the gene and the promoter methylation levels that were observed were particularly low. As the presence of early-life adversity was not assessed in this study, the findings in suicide completers may be mediated by different molecular pathways in the absence of early-life adversity.

Brain-Derived Neurotrophic Factor Gene

Neurotrophins or neurotrophic factors have been gaining interest as candidate molecules to study in association with the development of psychopathology because of their role in neuronal survival and plasticity as well as the fact that they are expressed in the limbic areas of the brain, where emotions and related behaviours are processed. Of the major neurotrophic factors, brain-derived neurotrophic factor (BDNF), a neurotrophin involved in neuronal growth and development has been the major focus in studying psychiatric conditions such as depressive disorders and suicide [81–83].

The role of early-life adversity in the epigenetic regulation of the BDNF gene was first investigated in a rat model of maternal care. Roth et al. [84] studied the effect of repeatedly exposing pups for short periods of time to non-biological mothers exhibiting abusive maternal behaviours, including pup avoidance and rough pup handling. Compared to controls, site-specific hypermethylation was found in the promoter region of transcripts IV and IX and decreased BDNF expression in the prefrontal cortex of the adult rats from the maltreated group. In addition, the deficits in BDNF expression were reversed by intracerebroventricular injection of a DNMT inhibitor, supporting the involvement of epigenetic mechanisms in the regulation of BDNF expression.

There have also been several investigations into the methylation of BDNF conducted on human tissues. Keller et al. [85] assessed, in post-mortem brain tissues from suicide completers, the methylation levels in a region encompassing part of non-coding exon IV and its promoter in the Wernicke area and found that methylation in four CpGs located downstream from the promoter IV transcription initiation site were significantly increased in suicide completers compared to controls. The methylation state of the BDNF gene was characterized in human peripheral blood leukocytes from borderline personality patients who were assessed for childhood maltreatment [86].

In this population of patients, peripheral levels of methylation in the BDNF gene promoter increased as a function of the number of childhood traumas experienced, suggesting that methylation of BDNF is associated with early-life adversity. Another recent study investigated BDNF methylation levels in blood samples obtained from patients being treated for major depressive disorder who were also assessed for suicidal behaviours [87]. Here, the investigators reported that greater methylation of the BDNF promoter was significantly correlated with a history of suicidal attempts and suicidal ideation. In addition, the level of BDNF methylation predicted the likelihood of improvement from suicidal ideation during treatment period such that patients with higher levels of BDNF methylation showed less improvement on suicide ideation compared to those with lower levels of BDNF methylation.

Serotoninergic Genes

Largely implicated in major depressive disorders and behavioural regulation, the serotonin system has also been studied in relation to epigenetic changes associated with early-life adversity and suicide. These alterations include lower concentration, binding, neurotransmission, and reuptake of serotonin and its metabolites associated with suicidality and major depression [88, 89]. The serotonin receptor subtype 2A (5-HT_{2A}) and its gene have been largely investigated in association studies of suicidal behaviour [90, 91] and, in particular, the 102 C/T polymorphism has been commonly investigated [92, 93]. Although methylation in the C allele variant in this polymorphism is associated with higher DNMT1 expression [94], increased methylation of this variant was detected in leukocytes from suicide ideators and a non-significant decrease in methylation was reported in the prefrontal cortex of suicide completers carrying the C allele [95]. These results suggest that methylation patterns may be different between individuals who committed suicide and those planning suicide.

The serotonin transporter (5-HTT) gene, among other things, has been implicated in the interaction between early-life stress and the risk of depression in human and primate models [96]. An early study analysing peripheral blood samples from Rhesus macaques found increased methylation of the 5-HTT gene promoter to be associated with increased reactivity to stress in maternally deprived, but not mother-reared, infants [97]. Associations between early-life adversity and DNA methylation of the 5-HTT gene were also reported in humans. A significant association between childhood sexual abuse and overall DNA methylation of the 5-HTT gene promoter region was reported in an investigation of lymphoblast DNA samples from subjects of the Iowa Adoption Study [98, 99]. In addition, the DNA methylation patterns observed in this gene were associated with the emergence of antisocial personality disorder in adulthood [98]. Another study using the same cohort of subjects also reported a correlation between childhood abuse and lymphoblast DNA methylation at 4 CpG sites in the non-promoter regions of the 5-HTT gene [100]. The methylation status of the 5-HTT promoter was examined in peripheral blood samples of patients with major depressive disorders and this was found to be significantly higher in those who experienced early-life adversity [101]. On the other hand, a more recent study conducted in peripheral blood from a German cohort failed to detect any site-specific changes in methylation associated with childhood trauma [102]. The discrepancy in findings among different studies may have been due to the difference in the type of cells investigated and promoter subregions examined as well as the method used to measure methylation, which are important to take into consideration when making comparisons.

Genome-Wide Epigenetic Changes

The studies described above have all focused on the epigenetic changes occurring on a specific gene but it is possible that early-life adversity may induce epigenetic changes across the whole genome. Labonté et al. [103] were the first to perform a genome-wide investigation of promoter DNA methylation in post-mortem hippocampal tissue collected from individuals with a history of severe childhood abuse. Methylation profiles were compared between individuals who experienced severe child abuse and non-abused controls and a total of 362 promoters were found to be differentially methylated in the abused group – 248 were hypermethylated while 114 were hypomethylated. Furthermore, the most significant DNA methylation changes occurred mainly in neurons and specifically in genes that are implicated in neural plasticity. A more recent genome-wide DNA methylation study in post-mortem ventral prefrontal cortex tissues obtained from individuals suffering from major depression who died by suicide examined 15,249 CpG sites and observed 8 times more CpG sites exhibiting increased methylation in the suicide group compared to controls. Moreover, the CpG sites that were hypermethylated in the depressed suicide group were located within genes implicated in behaviour, cell cycle, cell death and survival, and cellular and embryonic development [104]. Although these individuals were not assessed for the presence of early-life adversity, the findings combined with those from Labonté et al. [103] suggest that DNA hypermethylation in the brain may be a common feature associated with suicide.

There have been several genome-wide studies conducted in peripheral samples from individuals who experienced childhood maltreatment. Although these studies did not investigate suicidal behaviour, they addressed the epigenetic regulation of early-life adversity. Studying peripheral blood samples obtained from posttraumatic stress disorder patients, Mehta et al. [105] reported significant differences in the expression of several genes accompanied by greater instances of DNA methylation profile differences in the same genes in those who experienced childhood abuse than those without such histories. Another study examined genome-wide promoter DNA methylation in peripheral blood from subjects of the 1958 British cohort and found that childhood abuse was associated with significant differential methylation in 997 gene promoters – with 311 that were hypermethylated and 686 that were hypomethylated [106]. The methylation differences were overrepresented in genes implicated in key cell signalling pathways related to transcriptional regulation and development. In addition, this investigation revealed significant DNA methylation differences in several genes that code for microRNAs in subjects with histories of child abuse compared to those without. A genome-wide investigation of DNA methylation in saliva samples obtained from abused or neglected children revealed that 2,868 CpG sites were significantly differentially methylated in maltreated children compared to controls [107]. The CpG sites implicated were located within genes purported to be involved not only in psychiatric disorders but also in several other health conditions commonly associated with childhood abuse, including heart disease, stroke and respiratory disorders, among others. Altogether, these findings suggest that childhood abuse is associated with numerous epigenetic adaptations within the entire genome.

Conclusion

In this chapter, we have reviewed findings to suggest that early-life adversity, and in particular childhood abuse, affects molecular mechanisms involved in the regulation of emotion and behaviour. These effects include alterations in epigenetic regulation, which, by acting on genes involved in critical neuronal processes, is believed to be capable of inducing behavioural changes during development or later in life. Indeed, several environmentally induced epigenetic changes in the regulatory regions of genes implicated in the stress response, neuroplasticity and neurotransmission are observed in individuals who committed suicide and had histories of childhood abuse. These findings suggest that epigenetics may be a mechanism through which early environmental factors can induce long-term changes in behavioural responses and these changes could have a negative impact leading to the increased risk of suicide.

References

1 Turecki G, Ernst C, Jollant F, Labonte B, Mechawar N: The neurodevelopmental origins of suicidal behavior. Trends Neurosci 2012;35:14–23.
2 Brezo J, Paris J, Tremblay R, Vitaro F, Hebert M, Turecki G: Identifying correlates of suicide attempts in suicidal ideators: a population-based study. Psychol Med 2007;37:1551–1562.
3 Brezo J, Paris J, Barker ED, Tremblay R, Vitaro F, Zoccolillo M, et al: Natural history of suicidal behaviors in a population-based sample of young adults. Psychol Med 2007;37:1563–1574.
4 Fergusson DM, Woodward LJ, Horwood LJ: Risk factors and life processes associated with the onset of suicidal behaviour during adolescence and early adulthood. Psychol Med 2000;30:23–39.
5 Fergusson DM, Boden JM, Horwood LJ: Exposure to childhood sexual and physical abuse and adjustment in early adulthood. Child Abuse Negl 2008;32:607–619.
6 Brezo J, Paris J, Vitaro F, Hebert M, Tremblay RE, Turecki G: Predicting suicide attempts in young adults with histories of childhood abuse. Br J Psychiatry 2008;193:134–139.
7 Cutajar MC, Mullen PE, Ogloff JR, Thomas SD, Wells DL, Spataro J: Suicide and fatal drug overdose in child sexual abuse victims: a historical cohort study. Med J Aust 2010;192:184–187.

8 Martin G, Bergen HA, Richardson AS, Roeger L, Allison S: Sexual abuse and suicidality: gender differences in a large community sample of adolescents. Child Abuse Negl 2004;28:491–503.

9 Plunkett A, O'Toole B, Swanston H, Oates RK, Shrimpton S, Parkinson P: Suicide risk following child sexual abuse. Ambul Pediatr 2001;1:262–266.

10 Fanous AH, Prescott CA, Kendler KS: The prediction of thoughts of death or self-harm in a population-based sample of female twins. Psychol Med 2004;34:301–312.

11 Juon HS, Ensminger ME: Childhood, adolescent, and young adult predictors of suicidal behaviors: a prospective study of African Americans. J Child Psychol Psychiatry 1997;38:553–563.

12 Galera C, Bouvard MP, Encrenaz G, Messiah A, Fombonne E: Hyperactivity-inattention symptoms in childhood and suicidal behaviors in adolescence: the Youth Gazel Cohort. Acta Psychiatr Scand 2008; 118:480–489.

13 Evans E, Hawton K, Rodham K: Suicidal phenomena and abuse in adolescents: a review of epidemiological studies. Child Abuse Negl 2005;29:45–58.

14 Molnar BE, Berkman LF, Buka SL: Psychopathology, childhood sexual abuse and other childhood adversities: relative links to subsequent suicidal behaviour in the US. Psychol Med 2001;31:965–977.

15 Santa Mina EE, Gallop RM: Childhood sexual and physical abuse and adult self-harm and suicidal behaviour: a literature review. Can J Psychiatry 1998; 43:793–800.

16 Heim C, Nemeroff CB: The role of childhood trauma in the neurobiology of mood and anxiety disorders: preclinical and clinical studies. Biol Psychiatry 2001; 49:1023–1039.

17 Kendler KS, Bulik CM, Silberg J, Hettema JM, Myers J, Prescott CA: Childhood sexual abuse and adult psychiatric and substance use disorders in women: an epidemiological and cotwin control analysis. Arch Gen Psychiatry 2000;57:953–959.

18 Kaplan MJ, Klinetob NA: Childhood emotional trauma and chronic posttraumatic stress disorder in adult outpatients with treatment-resistant depression. J Nerv Ment Dis 2000;188:596–601.

19 Kendler KS, Kuhn JW, Prescott CA: Childhood sexual abuse, stressful life events and risk for major depression in women. Psychol Med 2004;34:1475–1482.

20 Agid O, Shapira B, Zislin J, Ritsner M, Hanin B, Murad H, et al: Environment and vulnerability to major psychiatric illness: a case control study of early parental loss in major depression, bipolar disorder and schizophrenia. Mol Psychiatry 1999;4:163–172.

21 Fergusson DM, Horwood LJ, Lynskey MT: Childhood sexual abuse and psychiatric disorder in young adulthood. II. Psychiatric outcomes of childhood sexual abuse. J Am Acad Child Adolesc Psychiatry 1996;35:1365–1374.

22 Labonte B, Turecki G: The epigenetics of suicide: explaining the biological effects of early life environmental adversity. Arch Suicide Res 2010;14:291–310.

23 Nagy C, Turecki G: Sensitive periods in epigenetics: bringing us closer to complex behavioral phenotypes. Epigenomics 2012;4:445–457.

24 Petronis A: Epigenetics as a unifying principle in the aetiology of complex traits and diseases. Nature 2010;465:721–727.

25 Hata K, Okano M, Lei H, Li E: Dnmt3L cooperates with the Dnmt3 family of de novo DNA methyltransferases to establish maternal imprints in mice. Development 2002;129:1983–1993.

26 Okano M, Xie S, Li E: Cloning and characterization of a family of novel mammalian DNA (cytosine-5) methyltransferases. Nat Genet 1998;19:219–220.

27 Lutz PE, Turecki G: DNA methylation and childhood maltreatment: from animal models to human studies. Neuroscience 2014;264:142–156.

28 Tahiliani M, Koh KP, Shen Y, Pastor WA, Bandukwala H, Brudno Y, et al: Conversion of 5-methylcytosine to 5-hydroxymethylcytosine in mammalian DNA by MLL partner TET1. Science 2009;324:930–935.

29 Ito S, D'Alessio AC, Taranova OV, Hong K, Sowers LC, Zhang Y: Role of Tet proteins in 5mC to 5hmC conversion, ES-cell self-renewal and inner cell mass specification. Nature 2010;466:1129–1133.

30 Nestor CE, Ottaviano R, Reddington J, Sproul D, Reinhardt D, Dunican D, et al: Tissue type is a major modifier of the 5-hydroxymethylcytosine content of human genes. Genome Res 2012;22:467–477.

31 Clements A, Poux AN, Lo WS, Pillus L, Berger SL, Marmorstein R: Structural basis for histone and phosphohistone binding by the GCN5 histone acetyltransferase. Mol Cell 2003;12:461–473.

32 Fischle W, Tseng BS, Dormann HL, Ueberheide BM, Garcia BA, Shabanowitz J, et al: Regulation of HP1-chromatin binding by histone H3 methylation and phosphorylation. Nature 2005;438:1116–1122.

33 Nelson CJ, Santos-Rosa H, Kouzarides T: Proline isomerization of histone H3 regulates lysine methylation and gene expression. Cell 2006;126:905–916.

34 Pray-Grant MG, Daniel JA, Schieltz D, Yates JR 3rd, Grant PA: Chd1 chromodomain links histone H3 methylation with SAGA- and SLIK-dependent acetylation. Nature 2005;433:434–438.

35 Santos-Rosa H, Schneider R, Bernstein BE, Karabetsou N, Morillon A, Weise C, et al: Methylation of histone H3 K4 mediates association of the Isw1p ATPase with chromatin. Mol Cell 2003;12:1325–1332.

36 Wysocka J, Swigut T, Milne TA, Dou Y, Zhang X, Burlingame AL, et al: WDR5 associates with histone H3 methylated at K4 and is essential for H3 K4 methylation and vertebrate development. Cell 2005;121:859–872.
37 Wysocka J, Swigut T, Xiao H, Milne TA, Kwon SY, Landry J, et al: A PHD finger of NURF couples histone H3 lysine 4 trimethylation with chromatin remodelling. Nature 2006;442:86–90.
38 Tsankova N, Renthal W, Kumar A, Nestler EJ: Epigenetic regulation in psychiatric disorders. Nat Rev Neurosci 2007;8:355–367.
39 Kirmizis A, Santos-Rosa H, Penkett CJ, Singer MA, Vermeulen M, Mann M, et al: Arginine methylation at histone H3R2 controls deposition of H3K4 trimethylation. Nature 2007;449:928–932.
40 Salcedo-Amaya AM, van Driel MA, Alako BT, Trelle MB, van den Elzen AM, Cohen AM, et al: Dynamic histone H3 epigenome marking during the intraerythrocytic cycle of *Plasmodium falciparum*. Proc Natl Acad Sci U S A 2009;106:9655–9660.
41 Barrera LO, Li Z, Smith AD, Arden KC, Cavenee WK, Zhang MQ, et al: Genome-wide mapping and analysis of active promoters in mouse embryonic stem cells and adult organs. Genome Res 2008;18:46–59.
42 Pokholok DK, Harbison CT, Levine S, Cole M, Hannett NM, Lee TI, et al: Genome-wide map of nucleosome acetylation and methylation in yeast. Cell 2005;122:517–527.
43 Wang Z, Zang C, Rosenfeld JA, Schones DE, Barski A, Cuddapah S, et al: Combinatorial patterns of histone acetylations and methylations in the human genome. Nat Genet 2008;40:897–903.
44 Xiao T, Shibata Y, Rao B, Laribee RN, O'Rourke R, Buck MJ, et al: The RNA polymerase II kinase Ctk1 regulates positioning of a 5′ histone methylation boundary along genes. Mol Cell Biol 2007;27:721–731.
45 Barski A, Cuddapah S, Cui K, Roh TY, Schones DE, Wang Z, et al: High-resolution profiling of histone methylations in the human genome. Cell 2007;129:823–837.
46 Bannister AJ, Zegerman P, Partridge JF, Miska EA, Thomas JO, Allshire RC, et al: Selective recognition of methylated lysine 9 on histone H3 by the HP1 chromo domain. Nature. 2001;410:120–124.
47 Botuyan MV, Lee J, Ward IM, Kim JE, Thompson JR, Chen J, et al: Structural basis for the methylation state-specific recognition of histone H4-K20 by 53BP1 and Crb2 in DNA repair. Cell 2006;127:1361–1373.
48 Lan F, Bayliss PE, Rinn JL, Whetstine JR, Wang JK, Chen S, et al: A histone H3 lysine 27 demethylase regulates animal posterior development. Nature 2007;449:689–694.
49 Nielsen SJ, Schneider R, Bauer UM, Bannister AJ, Morrison A, O'Carroll D, et al: Rb targets histone H3 methylation and HP1 to promoters. Nature 2001;412:561–565.
50 Sanders SL, Portoso M, Mata J, Bahler J, Allshire RC, Kouzarides T: Methylation of histone H4 lysine 20 controls recruitment of Crb2 to sites of DNA damage. Cell 2004;119:603–614.
51 Swigut T, Wysocka J: H3K27 demethylases, at long last. Cell 2007;131:29–32.
52 Smalheiser NR, Lugli G, Rizavi HS, Zhang H, Torvik VI, Pandey GN, et al: MicroRNA expression in rat brain exposed to repeated inescapable shock: differential alterations in learned helplessness vs. non-learned helplessness. Int J Neuropsychopharmacol 2011;14:1315–1325.
53 O'Connor RM, Dinan TG, Cryan JF: Little things on which happiness depends: microRNAs as novel therapeutic targets for the treatment of anxiety and depression. Mol Psychiatry 2012;17:359–376.
54 Omran A, Elimam D, Shalaby S, Peng J, Yin F. MicroRNAs: a light into the 'black box' of neuropediatric diseases? Neuromolecular Med 2012;14:244–261.
55 Saetrom P, Snove O Jr, Rossi JJ: Epigenetics and microRNAs. Pediatr Res 2007;61:17R–23R.
56 Heim C, Newport DJ, Mletzko T, Miller AH, Nemeroff CB: The link between childhood trauma and depression: insights from HPA axis studies in humans. Psychoneuroendocrinology 2008;33:693–710.
57 Pariante CM, Lightman SL: The HPA axis in major depression: classical theories and new developments. Trends Neurosci 2008;31:464–468.
58 Bremner JD, Randall P, Vermetten E, Staib L, Bronen RA, Mazure C, et al: Magnetic resonance imaging-based measurement of hippocampal volume in posttraumatic stress disorder related to childhood physical and sexual abuse – a preliminary report. Biol Psychiatry 1997;41:23–32.
59 Stein MB, Koverola C, Hanna C, Torchia MG, McClarty B: Hippocampal volume in women victimized by childhood sexual abuse. Psychol Med 1997;27:951–959.
60 Driessen M, Herrmann J, Stahl K, Zwaan M, Meier S, Hill A, et al: Magnetic resonance imaging volumes of the hippocampus and the amygdala in women with borderline personality disorder and early traumatization. Arch Gen Psychiatry 2000;57:1115–1122.
61 Carrion VG, Weems CF, Eliez S, Patwardhan A, Brown W, Ray RD, et al: Attenuation of frontal asymmetry in pediatric posttraumatic stress disorder. Biol Psychiatry 2001;50:943–951.
62 De Bellis MD, Keshavan MS, Frustaci K, Shifflett H, Iyengar S, Beers SR, et al: Superior temporal gyrus volumes in maltreated children and adolescents with PTSD. Biol Psychiatry 2002;51:544–552.

63 Bremner JD, Vythilingam M, Vermetten E, Southwick SM, McGlashan T, Nazeer A, et al: MRI and PET study of deficits in hippocampal structure and function in women with childhood sexual abuse and posttraumatic stress disorder. Am J Psychiatry 2003;160:924–932.
64 Heim C, Newport DJ, Heit S, Graham YP, Wilcox M, Bonsall R, et al: Pituitary-adrenal and autonomic responses to stress in women after sexual and physical abuse in childhood. JAMA 2000;284:592–597.
65 Heim C, Mletzko T, Purselle D, Musselman DL, Nemeroff CB: The dexamethasone/corticotropin-releasing factor test in men with major depression: role of childhood trauma. Biol Psychiatry 2008;63:398–405.
66 Carpenter LL, Tyrka AR, McDougle CJ, Malison RT, Owens MJ, Nemeroff CB, et al: Cerebrospinal fluid corticotropin-releasing factor and perceived early-life stress in depressed patients and healthy control subjects. Neuropsychopharmacology 2004;29:777–784.
67 Weaver IC, Cervoni N, Champagne FA, D'Alessio AC, Sharma S, Seckl JR, et al: Epigenetic programming by maternal behavior. Nat Neurosci 2004;7:847–854.
68 Meaney MJ: Maternal care, gene expression, and the transmission of individual differences in stress reactivity across generations. Annu Rev Neurosci 2001;24:1161–1192.
69 Higley JD, Hasert MF, Suomi SJ, Linnoila M: Nonhuman primate model of alcohol abuse: effects of early experience, personality, and stress on alcohol consumption. Proc Natl Acad Sci U S A 1991;88:7261–7265.
70 Levine A, Cohen D, Zadik Z: Urinary free cortisol values in children under stress. J Pediatr 1994;125:853–857.
71 Francis D, Diorio J, Liu D, Meaney MJ: Nongenomic transmission across generations of maternal behavior and stress responses in the rat. Science 1999;286:1155–1158.
72 Liu D, Diorio J, Tannenbaum B, Caldji C, Francis D, Freedman A, et al: Maternal care, hippocampal glucocorticoid receptors, and hypothalamic-pituitary-adrenal responses to stress. Science 1997;277:1659–1662.
73 McGowan PO, Sasaki A, D'Alessio AC, Dymov S, Labonte B, Szyf M, et al: Epigenetic regulation of the glucocorticoid receptor in human brain associates with childhood abuse. Nat Neurosci 2009;12:342–348.
74 Turner JD, Muller CP: Structure of the glucocorticoid receptor (NR3C1) gene 5′ untranslated region: identification, and tissue distribution of multiple new human exon 1. J Mol Endocrinol 2005;35:283–292.
75 Labonte B, Yerko V, Gross J, Mechawar N, Meaney MJ, Szyf M, et al: Differential glucocorticoid receptor exon 1_B, 1_C, and 1_H expression and methylation in suicide completers with a history of childhood abuse. Biol Psychiatry 2012;72:41–48.
76 Radtke KM, Ruf M, Gunter HM, Dohrmann K, Schauer M, Meyer A, et al: Transgenerational impact of intimate partner violence on methylation in the promoter of the glucocorticoid receptor. Transl Psychiatry 2011;1:1–6.
77 Tyrka AR, Price LH, Marsit C, Walters OC, Carpenter LL: Childhood adversity and epigenetic modulation of the leukocyte glucocorticoid receptor: preliminary findings in healthy adults. PLoS One 2012;7:e30148.
78 Perroud N, Dayer A, Piguet C, Nallet A, Favre S, Malafosse A, et al: Childhood maltreatment and methylation of the glucocorticoid receptor gene NR3C1 in bipolar disorder. Br J Psychiatry 2014;204:30–35.
79 Perroud N, Paoloni-Giacobino A, Prada P, Olie E, Salzmann A, Nicastro R, et al: Increased methylation of glucocorticoid receptor gene (NR3C1) in adults with a history of childhood maltreatment: a link with the severity and type of trauma. Transl Psychiatry 2011;1:e59.
80 Alt SR, Turner JD, Klok MD, Meijer OC, Lakke EA, Derijk RH, et al: Differential expression of glucocorticoid receptor transcripts in major depressive disorder is not epigenetically programmed. Psychoneuroendocrinology 2010;35:544–556.
81 Brunoni AR, Lopes M, Fregni F: A systematic review and meta-analysis of clinical studies on major depression and BDNF levels: implications for the role of neuroplasticity in depression. Int J Neuropsychopharmacol 2008;11:1169–1180.
82 Dwivedi Y, Rizavi HS, Conley RR, Roberts RC, Tamminga CA, Pandey GN: Altered gene expression of brain-derived neurotrophic factor and receptor tyrosine kinase B in postmortem brain of suicide subjects. Arch Gen Psychiatry 2003;60:804–815.
83 Pandey GN, Ren X, Rizavi HS, Conley RR, Roberts RC, Dwivedi Y: Brain-derived neurotrophic factor and tyrosine kinase B receptor signalling in postmortem brain of teenage suicide victims. Int J Neuropsychopharmacol 2008;11:1047–1061.
84 Roth TL, Lubin FD, Funk AJ, Sweatt JD: Lasting epigenetic influence of early-life adversity on the BDNF gene. Biol Psychiatry 2009;65:760–769.
85 Keller S, Sarchiapone M, Zarrilli F, Videtic A, Ferraro A, Carli V, et al: Increased BDNF promoter methylation in the Wernicke area of suicide subjects. Arch Gen Psychiatry 2010;67:258–267.

86 Perroud N, Salzmann A, Prada P, Nicastro R, Hoeppli ME, Furrer S, et al: Response to psychotherapy in borderline personality disorder and methylation status of the BDNF gene. Transl Psychiatry 2013;3:e207.
87 Kang HJ, Kim JM, Lee JY, Kim SY, Bae KY, Kim SW, et al: BDNF promoter methylation and suicidal behavior in depressive patients. J Affect Disord 2013; 151:679–685.
88 Cronholm B, Asberg M, Montgomery S, Schalling D: Suicidal behaviour syndrome with low CSF 5-HIAA. Br Med J 1977;1:776.
89 Bhagwagar Z, Cowen PJ: 'It's not over when it's over': persistent neurobiological abnormalities in recovered depressed patients. Psychol Med 2008;38:307–313.
90 Du L, Faludi G, Palkovits M, Bakish D, Hrdina PD: Serotonergic genes and suicidality. Crisis 2001;22: 54–60.
91 Turecki G, Briere R, Dewar K, Antonetti T, Lesage AD, Seguin M, et al: Prediction of level of serotonin 2A receptor binding by serotonin receptor 2A genetic variation in postmortem brain samples from subjects who did or did not commit suicide. Am J Psychiatry 1999;156:1456–1458.
92 Du L, Bakish D, Lapierre YD, Ravindran AV, Hrdina PD: Association of polymorphism of serotonin 2A receptor gene with suicidal ideation in major depressive disorder. Am J Med Genet 2000;96:56–60.
93 De Luca V, Likhodi O, Kennedy JL, Wong AH: Differential expression and parent-of-origin effect of the 5-HT2A receptor gene C102T polymorphism: analysis of suicidality in schizophrenia and bipolar disorder. Am J Med Genet B Neuropsychiatr Genet 2007;144B:370–374.
94 Polesskaya OO, Aston C, Sokolov BP: Allele C-specific methylation of the 5-HT2A receptor gene: evidence for correlation with its expression and expression of DNA methylase DNMT1. J Neurosci Res 2006;83:362–373.
95 De Luca V, Viggiano E, Dhoot R, Kennedy JL, Wong AH: Methylation and QTDT analysis of the 5-HT2A receptor 102C allele: analysis of suicidality in major psychosis. J Psychiatr Res 2009;43:532–537.
96 Caspi A, Sugden K, Moffitt TE, Taylor A, Craig IW, Harrington H, et al: Influence of life stress on depression: moderation by a polymorphism in the 5-HTT gene. Science 2003;301:386–389.
97 Capitanio JP, Mendoza SP, Mason WA, Maninger N: Rearing environment and hypothalamic-pituitary-adrenal regulation in young rhesus monkeys (*Macaca mulatta*). Dev Psychobiol 2005;46:318–330.
98 Beach SR, Brody GH, Todorov AA, Gunter TD, Philibert RA: Methylation at 5HTT mediates the impact of child sex abuse on women's antisocial behavior: an examination of the Iowa adoptee sample. Psychosom Med 2011;73:83–87.
99 Beach SR, Brody GH, Todorov AA, Gunter TD, Philibert RA: Methylation at SLC6A4 is linked to family history of child abuse: an examination of the Iowa Adoptee sample. Am J Med Genet B Neuropsychiatr Genet 2010;153B:710–713.
100 Vijayendran M, Beach SR, Plume JM, Brody GH, Philibert RA: Effects of genotype and child abuse on DNA methylation and gene expression at the serotonin transporter. Front Psychiatry 2012;3:55.
101 Kang HJ, Kim JM, Stewart R, Kim SY, Bae KY, Kim SW, et al: Association of SLC6A4 methylation with early adversity, characteristics and outcomes in depression. Progr Neuropsychopharmacol Biol Psychiatry 2013;44:23–28.
102 Wankerl M, Miller R, Kirschbaum C, Hennig J, Stalder T, Alexander N: Effects of genetic and early environmental risk factors for depression on serotonin transporter expression and methylation profiles. Transl Psychiatry 2014;4:e402.
103 Labonté B, Suderman M, Maussion G, Navaro L, Yerko V, Mahar I, et al: Genome-wide epigenetic regulation by early-life trauma. Arch Gen Psychiatry 2012;69:722–731.
104 Haghighi F, Xin Y, Chanrion B, O'Donnell AH, Ge Y, Dwork AJ, et al: Increased DNA methylation in the suicide brain. Dialogues Clin Neurosci 2014;16: 430–438.
105 Mehta D, Klengel T, Conneely KN, Smith AK, Altmann A, Pace TW, et al: Childhood maltreatment is associated with distinct genomic and epigenetic profiles in posttraumatic stress disorder. Proc Nat Acad Sci USA 2013;110:8302–8307.
106 Suderman M, Borghol N, Pappas JJ, Pinto Pereira SM, Pembrey M, Hertzman C, et al: Childhood abuse is associated with methylation of multiple loci in adult DNA. BMC Med Genomics 2014;7:13.
107 Yang BZ, Zhang H, Ge W, Weder N, Douglas-Palumberi H, Perepletchikova F, et al: Child abuse and epigenetic mechanisms of disease risk. Am J Prev Med 2013;44:101–107.

Gustavo Turecki, MD, PhD
Douglas Mental Health University Institute
6875 LaSalle Blvd
Montreal, QC H4H 1R3 (Canada)
E-Mail gustavo.turecki@mcgill.ca

Kaschka WP, Rujescu D (eds): Biological Aspects of Suicidal Behavior.
Adv Biol Psychiatry. Basel, Karger, 2016, vol 30, pp 88–100 (DOI: 10.1159/000434739)

Neurocognitive Processes and Decision Making in Suicidal Behaviour

Stéphane Richard-Devantoy[a–c] • Philippe Courtet[d–f]

[a]Department of Psychiatry, McGill University, and [b]McGill Group for Suicide Studies, Douglas Mental Health University Institute, Montreal, Que., Canada; [c]Laboratoire de Psychologie des Pays de la Loire EA 4638, Université de Nantes et Angers, Angers, [d]Department of Emergency Psychiatry and Post-Acute Care, CHU Montpellier, and [e]Inserm U1061, Université Montpellier, Montpellier, and [f]Fondamental Foundation, Créteil, France

Abstract

Suicidal behaviour has been investigated at sociological, clinical, genetic, cellular, and molecular levels. More recently, neuropsychological and brain imaging studies have been conducted to improve our understanding of this complex behaviour. Here, we review the growing number of studies published in the neuropsychological field. A total of 68 studies were found, most of them investigating middle-aged adults. Findings generally support the concept of vulnerability to suicidal behaviour, which is associated with certain neuropsychological deficits: deficient decision making, reduced cognitive control and verbal fluency and impairment of autobiographical (over-general and less specific), long-term and working memory. More studies are necessary to confirm these findings and increase our understanding of these heterogeneous behaviours. This may be a first step toward uncovering more powerful predictive markers and identifying more efficient therapeutic targets.

A Stress-Diathesis Model of Suicidal Behaviour

Suicide rates are especially elevated among those with mental disorders. Epidemiological studies have revealed a significantly increased likelihood of suicide among many psychiatric disorders, including but not limited to major depression, bipolar disorder, schizophrenia, and borderline personality disorder [1–3]. Moreover, postmortem studies reported the existence of mental disorders in more than 90% of cases of suicide [4]. However, more than 90% of individuals with mental disorder will never commit suicide [5], suggesting that mental disorder is not a sufficient condition for suicide.

Over the past decades, a large variety of studies have been conducted to support the concept of vulnerability at the neurobiological level, ranging from biochemical [6] to genetic/epigenetic [7, 8] and cell morphological studies [9–11]. The earliest and most replicated known biological risk factor associated with suicidal acts was a low 5-hydroxyindoleacetic acid (5-HIAA) level, the main metabolite of serotonin, in cerebrospinal fluid [12]. Subsequent studies in the area have also investigated serotonergic alterations in post-mortem studies [13] and the genetics of serotonin synthesis mechanisms (e.g. tryptophan hydroxylase) and transportation (e.g. serotonin transporter) [14, 15]. The general hypothesis derived from these findings is a deficient modulation of the prefrontal cortex and other brain regions by the serotonergic system, an alteration that may possess some trait-like characteristics, including long-term stability, and would underlie clinical and cognitive traits, including a higher propensity for impulsivity [16] or risky decision making [17]. Hypothalamic-pituitary-adrenal (HPA) axis sensitivity has also been implicated in suicidal behaviour [18]. Recent data suggest that the HPA response is also increased during an inhibition task in relatives of suicide completers [19], revealing another heritable biological trait. Serotonergic and HPA systems may synergistically contribute to suicidal behaviour [20].

A stress-diathesis model postulates a vulnerability to suicidal acts with genetic and early developmental components (including childhood abuse) interacting with proximal stressful events, e.g. social negative events like marital conflict or job loss, depression or alcohol abuse [21]. This lower ability to respond adequately to stress is also underlined by numerous studies showing deficient cognitive functioning, notably disadvantageous decision making [22, 23] or reduced cognitive inhibition [24]. Decision-making deficit has been found in normothymic patients (at a distance from their suicidal act) in comparison to patient controls, suggesting it represents a cognitive trait-marker of suicide vulnerability.

Although it may seem out of fashion nowadays in comparison to functional neuroimaging with which it shares the exploration of the thinking brain, neuropsychology has brought very relevant data to the understanding of the vulnerability to suicidal behaviour [25–26]. According to the latest meta-analyses and reviews, a series of replicated neuropsychological deficits has been demonstrated in patients with suicidal behaviour compared to controls [23]. Notable deficits include disadvantageous decision making (mainly measured by the Iowa gambling task) and reduced verbal fluency and cognitive control (measured by the Stroop task). See figure 1 for a summary of neuropsychological key players in suicide vulnerability.

Decision-Making Findings

Impaired decision making was found in non-depressed patients with a past history of suicidal acts (notably those who used a violent method) in comparison to non-depressed patients with no history of suicidal act and healthy controls [27–29]. Suicide

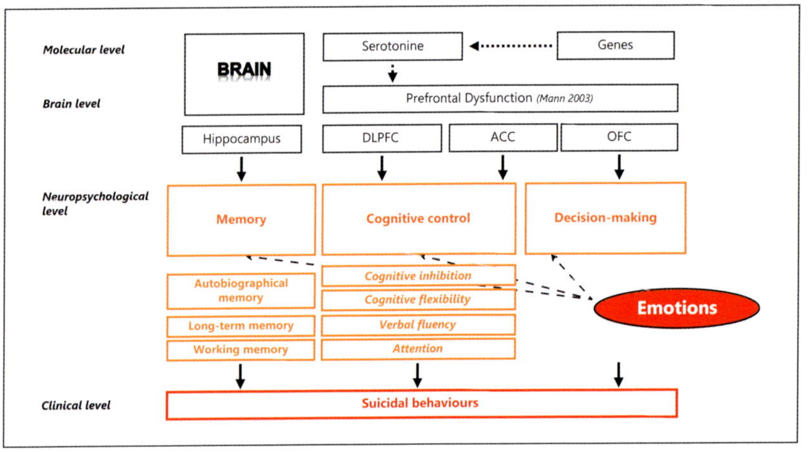

Fig. 1. Summary of neuropsychological key players in suicide vulnerability. ACC = Anterior cingulate cortex; DLPFC = dorsolateral prefrontal cortex; OFC = orbitofrontal cortex. Prefrontal dysfunction: see Mann [21], 2013.

attempters tend to choose options with higher immediate reward but long-term loss over options with lower reward but long-term gain, an impairment that is related to lateral orbitofrontal cortex dysfunction in this population [28]. This result in middle-aged patients has been replicated in studies with patients suffering from depressive [30] or bipolar disorder [31, 32] but not by other studies [33–35]. Interestingly, decision-making deficit was also found in both adolescent [36–40] and elderly [41–43] suicide attempters, suggesting that disadvantageous decision making could be a factor of cognitive vulnerability to suicidal behaviours across the lifespan. Decision-making impairment in suicide attempters was further correlated to the likelihood of interpersonal difficulties, a well-known trigger of suicidal acts, and with genetic variants previously related to suicidal behaviours [27, 44]. These findings point toward decision-making deficit being at the interface of genes and the (social) environment. Decision-making deficit could also be a potential endophenotype of suicidal behaviours, although to date there is a lack of information regarding stability of performance over time and deficits in healthy relatives [45]. Finally, it has been reported that decision-making impairment and deficient cognitive control do not show strong correlation [46], suggesting that they may synergistically, yet independently, contribute to suicidal behaviour.

Cognitive Control Findings

Cognitive Flexibility

Initial reports suggested more cognitive rigidity in suicide attempters [47], a result that has not always been replicated, notably during remission from the suicidal crisis

[48]. More recently, cognitive inflexibility has been demonstrated in depressed middle-aged suicide attempters [49, 50] and ideators [51] and in old-age suicide attempters [52]. It was found to be more pronounced when suicidal intent was high [49]. In adolescent suicide attempters, cognitive inflexibility measured by perseverative errors on the Wisconsin card-sorting test predicted suicidal ideation at the 6-month follow-up [53]. A recent study showed that cognitive inflexibility may be found in healthy relatives of suicide completers [54], suggesting the heritability of this cognitive trait. Cognitive inflexibility may render individuals less likely to adapt to changing environment and, therefore, more likely to experience distress in these conditions.

Verbal Fluency

Reduced verbal fluency has been found in depressed suicide attempters [49, 55], presenting a bipolar I disorder but not a bipolar II disorder [56]. This was not observed in depressed subjects with current suicidal ideation [51]. Impairment in letter fluency was higher in high-lethality compared to low-lethality suicide attempters [49]. In elderly people, results were more contradictory [50, 57]. A deficit in verbal fluency may indirectly represent the inability of suicide attempters to communicate their difficulties to others, a process that may facilitate the committing of the act.

Cognitive Inhibition

Several studies suggest a deficit of cognitive inhibition in suicide attempters [49, 56, 58] and ideators [30] using the Stroop test or a go/no-go test, while others could not find any deficit [31, 51]. Importantly, cognitive inhibition impairment was increased in an emotional context [59–61]. For instance, compared to controls, suicide attempters took longer to read the colour of suicide-related [59–61] and negative words [59] in a modified version of the Stroop test. Similarly, a social stress test increased inhibition deficit in relatives of suicide completers in comparison to relatives of depressed patients [62], underlying both the transmission of cognitive deficits and the impact of emotions. All aspects of cognitive inhibition (access, suppression and restraint) were shown to be impaired in elderly depressed suicide attempters versus patients and healthy controls [63]. In another study, high-lethality elderly depressed attempters took longer to complete the inhibition condition of the task compared to depressed control subjects, healthy control subjects and suicide ideators, except low-lethality attempters, who demonstrated an intermediate performance [64]. This difference remained after taking into account possible confounders, including education, global cognitive performance and information processing speed. Interestingly, low-lethality suicide attempters tended to make more uncorrected errors in all conditions, suggesting a careless approach to the task or a lack of monitoring. These results indicate that people with a history of attempted suicide display a considerable cognitive heterogeneity, which can be parsed to some extent by grouping them into high- versus low-lethality attempters [49, 65, 66].

Attention

Deficits of attention were found to be significantly higher in depressed subjects with a past history of suicidal behaviour [58, 67], especially those with high suicidal intent [68] and those who committed multiple suicide attempts [69]. A deficit in attentional control may contribute to a variety of cognitive deficits in suicidal patients, although it does not seem to be a causal factor of decision-making impairment.

Memory Findings

The first meta-analysis on mnesic functions associated with the vulnerability to suicidal behaviour revealed interesting findings [26]. Overall, three domains (autobiographical memory reported as being over-general and less specific, long-term memory and working memory) were found to be altered in suicide attempters versus patient controls and in patient controls versus healthy controls, suggesting greater alterations in those with a vulnerability to suicidal behaviour than in those with comorbid disorders but no history of suicidality. One domain (short-term memory) was only altered in the comparison between patient control groups and healthy controls, suggesting that impairment in this domain is mostly related to related psychiatric disorders (in this case, mainly major depression). Finally, no memory alteration was found to be specifically associated with the vulnerability to suicidal behaviour (in the contrast between suicide attempters and both patient and healthy control groups but not between patient and healthy controls).

Among 14 studies, 8 reported less specific and more general autobiographical memories in suicide attempters compared to patient [70–75] and healthy controls [71–74, 76] across different age and diagnosis groups; 1 study in psychosis reported the opposite results [77] and 1 study reported no between-group difference [78]. Finally, 4 studies reported a significant association between poor performance in autobiographical memory and a higher number of suicide attempts [79–82], especially in those with an early age of onset of history of childhood abuse [79].

Among 10 studies on working memory, no differences between suicide attempters and patient controls were found in 5 studies; 4 studies reported worse performances in suicide attempters with mood disorder [83–86]. In 1 study [83], high-lethality attempters were found to outperform low-lethality attempters, although it is not clear whether this result is a true-positive result or whether it is related to the high frequency of violent attempters in the low-lethality group or to a sampling bias. In addition, 1 study showed better performance in suicide attempters with schizophrenia [87] relative to patient controls.

No between-group differences in short-term memory were found in 10 studies but 2 studies in schizophrenia found better performances in suicide attempters compared to patient controls [87, 88] and 3 studies in mood disorders found worse performance in suicide attempters, especially in high-lethality attempters [83, 89, 90].

Similarly, 3 studies found no between-group differences in long-term memory but 2 studies in schizophrenia found better performances in suicide attempters compared to patient controls [87, 91] and 3 studies in mood disorders found worse performance in suicide attempters, especially in high-lethality attempters [83, 89, 90].

Discussion

It is becoming increasingly clear that individuals who attempt suicide or die by suicide have a predisposition for this behaviour [92, 93]. In addition to impulsive aggression [94] and persistent hopelessness [95, 96], several studies have now reported impairments in cognitive domains such as autobiographical (over-general and less specific), long-term and working memory [26], as well as decision making, verbal fluency and cognitive control [26].

In fact, neurocognitive vulnerability to suicide behaviour may be modulated by sociodemographic factors (age and gender), diagnosis (depression, bipolar disorder, schizophrenia, personality disorder…) characteristics of the suicide attempters and at least the lethality of the suicidal act. Indeed, studies of neuropsychological components of suicide vulnerability examined various populations. For example, some enrolled only adolescents [40], middle-aged [83] or elderly [85] participants. Some studies were only conducted in males [28], while most included both genders.

In addition, some studies included only patients with bipolar depression [31], with a unipolar depressive disorder [30] or a combination of patients with both subtypes of mood disorder [29]. Also, some studies were conducted in patients who were acutely depressed [85, 97], while others focused on those in remission [29]. A recent study demonstrated that suicide attempters performed more poorly in attention, memory and working memory domains independently of current depressive symptomatology [98].

In the case of schizophrenia patients, 5 studies showed contradictory results. In 2 studies, outpatient suicide attempters with schizophrenia tended to outperform schizophrenic non-attempters in executive functioning, namely on measures of attention and verbal fluency [88], and cognitive flexibility [87, 88]. However, the 3 other studies did not find any group difference in executive performances [91, 99, 100].

In the case of bipolar disorder, results are contradictory. For example, severe suicide attempters outperformed non-severe attempters in verbal learning and non-attempters in the Stroop word reading part [101]. Besides, the literature has suggested that suicidal behaviour and bipolar disorder appear to share vulnerability factors, endophenotypes and susceptibility genes, which may explain the high suicide risk associated with this disorder [102]. For example, decision-making impairment, a cognitive trait associated with suicidal behaviour, has been reported in patients with bipolar disorder [33], especially if suicidal [32].

Moreover, suicide attempts vary in medical severity, from acts that cause no medical damage to those that would be fatal without rescue. There is increasing evidence that the cognitive and broader biological profile of those individuals who make serious (high-lethality) versus low-lethality suicide attempts are different [43, 49, 66, 90, 103]. It has been previously reported that, in an overlapping sample of older people with depression, a history of high-lethality attempts predicted poor performance on the Wisconsin card-sorting test [66]. In a US study of younger adults, Keilp et al. [83] found an impairment in Stroop performance in suicide attempters compared to both patient and healthy control subjects. The finding of Richard-Devantoy et al. [64] of a high uncorrected error rate in low-lethality attempters parallels that of a Brazilian study by Malloy-Diniz et al. [31], who reported a positive correlation between the number of suicide attempts and the number of errors on the Stroop test in younger bipolar I patients. Findings, however, are mixed with respect to the motor component of cognitive inhibition captured by the go/no-go test [83, 85, 86]. The study of cognitive inhibition in elderly suicide attempters [85] found significant impairments in access to relevant information and deletion of irrelevant information in comparison to both depressed and healthy control groups. The intermediate performance of suicide ideators in a recent paper [64] suggests a dose-response relationship between cognitive control deficits and the progression of the suicidal process. This dose-response relationship, however, was lacking in a previous analysis of a screening measure of cognitive control, EXIT25, in a larger overlapping sample of older adults [104], where suicide ideators performed as poorly as suicide attempters.

How exactly does poor cognitive control and decision-making contribute to suicidal behaviour? Cognitive control can be thought of as the ability to organize information in a way that helps achieve the best outcome. It underlies certain (but not all) aspects of decision making, which in turn appears impaired in younger [29] and older [42, 65] suicide attempters. Decisions that involve uncertainty, options with multiple features and changes over time place particularly high demands on cognitive control [105, 106]. Since the suicidal process involves the following: (1) a catastrophic accumulation of stressors, (2) an inability to find alternative solutions and (3) a disregard for the tragic consequences of suicide, future experiments need to elucidate the contribution of poor cognitive control to these failures of real-life problem solving and decision making. We propose the hypothesis that the inability to find and implement alternative solutions in a suicidal crisis is the most direct consequence of poor cognitive control.

Deficits of cognitive inhibition in suicidal patients may be related to the dysfunction of the lateral prefrontoparietal network [107–109]. Cognitive control abilities in general depend on the associative cortices comprising the lateral frontoparietal and cingulo-opercular networks [106, 110]. Studies have implicated that the dorsolateral prefrontal cortex is crucial in working memory processes and in the ability to inhibit responses [111, 112]. Indeed, initial results from FDG-PET [113] and fMRI studies [25] point to frontoparietal and cingulo-opercular alterations in attempted suicide. FDG-PET studies have found lower regional cerebral metabolic rates of glucose in right dorsolateral prefrontal regions of suicide attempters compared to depressed non-suicidal subjects [113]. Deficits in cognitive control and the putative frontoparietal and cingulo-opercular alterations in attempted suicide appear distinct from impairments in value-based decision making paralleled by paralimbic and particularly ventromedial prefrontal cortex dysfunction [114, 115] and the anterior cingulate cortex [115]. These latter deficits are illustrated by a recent finding of paralimbic and particularly ventromedial prefrontal cortex disruptions during value-based decision making in older suicide attempters, which correlated with high impulsivity, a neglect of decision-relevant information and poorly planned suicide attempts [116]. Thus, we would argue for the existence of two independent vulnerability pathways marked by cognitive control/frontoparietal versus value/paralimbic dysfunction. The first pathway, illustrated by the current behavioural findings, may involve an inability to find and implement alternative solutions in a crisis. The second, the value/paralimbic pathway, may involve impulsivity, a low threshold for suicidal acts and a disregard for deterrents.

Conclusion

Neuropsychological studies generally support the concept of vulnerability to suicidal behaviour, with some data suggesting the heritability of certain deficits. The suicidal crisis may result from both deficient value-based processes, facilitating the automatic triggering of an acute emotional state, and deficient regulatory processes, leading to ruminations, psychological pain, suicidal ideas, and in some, but not all patients, a suicidal act [25]. This model needs to be tested. Of note, little is known about gender or age differences in cognitive deficits related to suicidal behaviour.

In our opinion, neuropsychology, a much less expensive tool than neuroimaging, will remain a relevant investigation in the years to come for the understanding of suicidal behaviours, whereas its clinical application may still need more time, as for other biomarkers. Longitudinal studies will offer a glimpse into the true predictive power of neuropsychological tests. Finally, future studies should investigate how these findings may be used in intervention aimed at preventing suicide, which is the ultimate goal of suicide research.

References

1 Hawton K, van Heeringen K: Suicide. Lancet 2009; 373:1372–1381.
2 Arsenault-Lapierre G, Kim C, Turecki G: Psychiatric diagnoses in 3,275 suicides: a meta-analysis. BMC Psychiatry 2004;4:37.
3 Skodol AE, Gunderson JG, McGlashan TH, Dyck IR, Stout RL, Bender DS, et al: Functional impairment in patients with schizotypal, borderline, avoidant, or obsessive-compulsive personality disorder. Am J Psychiatry 2002;159:276–283.
4 Isometsa ET: Psychological autopsy studies – a review. Eur Psychiatry 2001;16:379–385.
5 Bostwick JM, Pankratz VS: Affective disorders and suicide risk: a reexamination. Am J Psychiatry 2000; 157:1925–1932.
6 Mann JJ, Currier D: A review of prospective studies of biologic predictors of suicidal behavior in mood disorders. Arch Suicide Res 2007;11:3–16.
7 Brent DA, Mann JJ: Family genetic studies, suicide, and suicidal behavior. Am J Med Genet C Semin Med Genet 2005;133C:13–24.
8 Fiori LM, Turecki G: Genetic and epigenetic influences on expression of spermine synthase and spermine oxidase in suicide completers. Int J Neuropsychopharmacol 2010;13:725–736.
9 Torres-Platas SG, Hercher C, Davoli MA, Maussion G, Labonte B, Turecki G, et al: Astrocytic hypertrophy in anterior cingulate white matter of depressed suicides. Neuropsychopharmacology 2011;36:2650–2658.
10 Hercher C, Turecki G, Mechawar N: Through the looking glass: examining neuroanatomical evidence for cellular alterations in major depression. J Psychiatr Res 2009;43:947–961.
11 Hercher C, Parent M, Flores C, Canetti L, Turecki G, Mechawar N: Alcohol dependence-related increase of glial cell density in the anterior cingulate cortex of suicide completers. J Psychiatry Neurosci 2009;34: 281–288.
12 Nordstrom P, Samuelsson M, Asberg M, Traskman-Bendz L, Aberg-Wistedt A, Nordin C, et al: CSF 5-HIAA predicts suicide risk after attempted suicide. Suicide Life Threat Behav 1994;24:1–9.
13 Mann JJ, Huang YY, Underwood MD, Kassir SA, Oppenheim S, Kelly TM, et al: A serotonin transporter gene promoter polymorphism (5-HTTLPR) and prefrontal cortical binding in major depression and suicide. Arch Gen Psychiatry 2000;57:729–738.
14 Courtet P, Jollant F, Castelnau D, Buresi C, Malafosse A: Suicidal behavior: relationship between phenotype and serotonergic genotype. Am J Med Genet C Semin Med Genet 2005;133C:25–33.
15 Courtet P, Picot MC, Bellivier F, Torres S, Jollant F, Michelon C, et al: Serotonin transporter gene may be involved in short-term risk of subsequent suicide attempts. Biol Psychiatry 2004;55:46–51.
16 Booij L, Swenne CA, Brosschot JF, Haffmans PM, Thayer JF, Van der Does AJ: Tryptophan depletion affects heart rate variability and impulsivity in remitted depressed patients with a history of suicidal ideation. Biol Psychiatry 2006;60:507–514.
17 Jollant F, Buresi C, Guillaume S, Jaussent I, Bellivier F, Leboyer M, et al: The influence of four serotonin-related genes on decision-making in suicide attempters. Am J Med Genet B Neuropsychiatr Genet 2007;144:615–624.
18 Coryell W: Do serum cholesterol values and DST results comprise independent risk factors for suicide? In Dwivedi Y (ed): The Neurobiological Basis of Suicide. Boca Raton, CRC Press, 2012.
19 McGirr A, Diaconu G, Berlim MT, Pruessner JC, Sable R, Cabot S, et al: Dysregulation of the sympathetic nervous system, hypothalamic-pituitary-adrenal axis and executive function in individuals at risk for suicide. J Psychiatry Neurosci 2010;35:399–408.
20 Caspi A, Sugden K, Moffitt TE, Taylor A, Craig IW, Harrington H, et al: Influence of life stress on depression: moderation by a polymorphism in the 5-HTT gene. Science 2003;301:386–389.
21 Mann JJ: Neurobiology of suicidal behaviour. Nat Rev Neurosci 2003;4:819–828.
22 Jollant F, Bellivier F, Leboyer M, Astruc B, Torres S, Verdier R, et al: Impaired decision making in suicide attempters. Am J Psychiatry 2005;162:304–310.
23 Richard-Devantoy S, Berlim MT, Jollant F: A meta-analysis of neuropsychological markers of vulnerability to suicidal behavior in mood disorders. Psychol Med 2014;44:1663–1673.
24 Richard-Devantoy S, Gorwood P, Annweiler C, Olie JP, Le Gall D, Beauchet O: Suicidal behaviours in affective disorders: a deficit of cognitive inhibition? Can J Psychiatry 2012;57:254–262.
25 Jollant F, Lawrence NL, Olie E, Guillaume S, Courtet P: The suicidal mind and brain: a review of neuropsychological and neuroimaging studies. World J Biol Psychiatry 2011;12:319–339.
26 Richard-Devantoy S, Berlim MT, Jollant F: Suicidal behaviour and memory: a systematic review and meta-analysis. World J Biol Psychiatry 2014, Epub ahead of print.
27 Jollant F, Guillaume S, Jaussent I, Castelnau D, Malafosse A, Courtet P: Impaired decision-making in suicide attempters may increase the risk of problems in affective relationships. J Affect Disord 2007;99:59–62.

28 Jollant F, Lawrence NS, Olie E, O'Daly O, Malafosse A, Courtet P, et al: Decreased activation of lateral orbitofrontal cortex during risky choices under uncertainty is associated with disadvantageous decision-making and suicidal behavior. Neuroimage 2010;51: 1275–1281.
29 Jollant F, Bellivier F, Leboyer M, Astruc B, Torres S, Verdier R, et al: Impaired decision making in suicide attempters. Am J Psychiatry 2005;162:304–310.
30 Westheide J, Quednow BB, Kuhn KU, Hoppe C, Cooper-Mahkorn D, Hawellek B, et al: Executive performance of depressed suicide attempters: the role of suicidal ideation. Eur Arch Psychiatry Clin Neurosci 2008;258:414–421.
31 Malloy-Diniz LF, Neves FS, Abrantes SS, Fuentes D, Correa H: Suicide behavior and neuropsychological assessment of type I bipolar patients. J Affect Disord 2009;112:231–236.
32 Martino DJ, Strejilevich SA, Torralva T, Manes F: Decision making in euthymic bipolar I and bipolar II disorders. Psychol Med 2011;41:1319–1327.
33 Adida M, Jollant F, Clark L, Besnier N, Guillaume S, Kaladjian A, et al: Trait-related decision-making impairment in the three phases of bipolar disorder. Biol Psychiatry 2011;70:357–365.
34 Gilbert AM, Garno JL, Braga RJ, Shaya Y, Goldberg TE, Malhotra AK, et al: Clinical and cognitive correlates of suicide attempts in bipolar disorder: is suicide predictable? J Clin Psychiatry 2011;72:1027–1033.
35 Gorlyn M, Keilp JG, Oquendo MA, Burke AK, John Mann J: Iowa gambling task performance in currently depressed suicide attempters. Psychiatry Res 2013; 207:150–157.
36 Dougherty DM, Mathias CW, Marsh-Richard DM, Prevette KN, Dawes MA, Hatzis ES, et al: Impulsivity and clinical symptoms among adolescents with non-suicidal self-injury with or without attempted suicide. Psychiatry Res 2009;169:22–27.
37 Mathias CW, Dougherty DM, James LM, Richard DM, Dawes MA, Acheson A, et al: Intolerance to delayed reward in girls with multiple suicide attempts. Suicide Life Threat Behav 2011;41:277–286.
38 Oldershaw A, Grima E, Jollant F, Richards C, Simic M, Taylor L, et al: Decision making and problem solving in adolescents who deliberately self-harm. Psychol Med 2009;39:95–104.
39 Ackerman JP, McBee-Strayer SM, Mendoza K, Stevens J, Sheftall AH, Campo JV, et al: Risk-sensitive decision-making deficit in adolescent suicide attempters. J Child Adolesc Psychopharmacol 2015; 25:109–113.
40 Bridge JA, McBee-Strayer SM, Cannon EA, Sheftall AH, Reynolds B, Campo JV, et al: Impaired decision making in adolescent suicide attempters. J Am Acad Child Adolesc Psychiatry 2012;51:394–403.
41 Clark L, Dombrovski AY, Siegle GJ, Butters MA, Shollenberger CL, Sahakian BJ, et al: Impairment in risk-sensitive decision-making in older suicide attempters with depression. Psychol Aging 2011;26: 321–330.
42 Dombrovski AY, Clark L, Siegle GJ, Butters MA, Ichikawa N, Sahakian BJ, et al: Reward/punishment reversal learning in older suicide attempters. Am J Psychiatry 2010;167:699–707.
43 Dombrovski AY, Szanto K, Siegle GJ, Wallace ML, Forman SD, Sahakian B, et al: Lethal forethought: delayed reward discounting differentiates high- and low-lethality suicide attempts in old age. Biol Psychiatry 2011;70:138–144.
44 Jollant F, Guillaume S, Jaussent I, Bellivier F, Leboyer M, Castelnau D, et al: Psychiatric diagnoses and personality traits associated with disadvantageous decision-making. Eur Psychiatry 2007;22:455–461.
45 Courtet P, Wyart M, Jaussent I, Ritchie K, Jollant F: Decision making and vulnerability to suicidal behaviour in elderly. Eur Psychiatry 2011;26:21–64.
46 Richard-Devantoy S, Olie E, Guillaume S, Bechara A, Courtet P, Jollant F: Distinct alterations in value-based decision-making and cognitive control in suicide attempters: toward a dual neurocognitive model. J Affect Disord 2013;151:1120–1124.
47 Neuringer C: Rigid thinking in suicidal individuals. J Consult Psychol 1964;28:54–58.
48 Perrah M, Wichman H: Cognitive rigidity in suicide attempters. Suicide Life Threat Behav 1987;17:251–255.
49 Keilp JG, Sackeim HA, Brodsky BS, Oquendo MA, Malone KM, Mann JJ: Neuropsychological dysfunction in depressed suicide attempters. Am J Psychiatry 2001;158:735–741.
50 King DA, Conwell Y, Cox C, Henderson RE, Denning DG, Caine ED: A neuropsychological comparison of depressed suicide attempters and nonattempters. J Neuropsychiatry Clin Neurosci 2000;12: 64–70.
51 Marzuk PM, Hartwell N, Leon AC, Portera L: Executive functioning in depressed patients with suicidal ideation. Acta Psychiatr Scand 2005;112:294–301.
52 McGirr A, Dombrovski AY, Butters MA, Clark L, Szanto K: Deterministic learning and attempted suicide among older depressed individuals: cognitive assessment using the Wisconsin card sorting task. J Psychiatr Res 2012;46:226–232.
53 Miranda R, Gallagher M, Bauchner B, Vaysman R, Marroquin B: Cognitive inflexibility as a prospective predictor of suicidal ideation among young adults with a suicide attempt history. Depress Anxiety 2012;29:180–186.
54 McGirr A, Jollant F, Turecki G: Neurocognitive alterations in first degree relatives of suicide completers. J Affect Disord 2013;145:264–269.

55 Bartfai A, Winborg IM, Nordstrom P, Asberg M: Suicidal behavior and cognitive flexibility: design and verbal fluency after attempted suicide. Suicide Life Threat Behav 1990;20:254–266.
56 Harkavy-Friedman JM, Keilp JG, Grunenbaum MF, Sher L, Printz D, Burke AK, et al: Are BPI and BPII suicide attempters distinct neuropsychologically? J Affect Disord 2006;94:255–259.
57 Dombrovski AY, Butters MA, Reynolds CF 3rd, Houck PR, Clark L, Mazumdar S, et al: Cognitive performance in suicidal depressed elderly: preliminary report. Am J Geriatr Psychiatry 2008;16:109–115.
58 Keilp JG, Gorlyn M, Oquendo MA, Burke AK, Mann JJ: Attention deficit in depressed suicide attempters. Psychiatry Res 2008;159:7–17.
59 Williams JM, Broadbent K: Distraction by emotional stimuli: use of a Stroop task with suicide attempters. Br J Clin Psychol 1986;25:101–110.
60 Becker ES, Strohbach D, Rinck M: A specific attentional bias in suicide attempters. J Nerv Ment Dis 1999;187:730–735.
61 Cha CB, Najmi S, Park JM, Finn CT, Nock MK: Attentional bias toward suicide-related stimuli predicts suicidal behavior. J Abnorm Psychol 2010;119:616–622.
62 McGirr A, Diaconu G, Berlim MT, Pruessner JC, Sable R, Cabot S, et al: Dysregulation of the sympathetic nervous system, hypothalamic-pituitary-adrenal axis and executive function in individuals at risk for suicide. J Psychiatry Neurosci 2010;35:399–408.
63 Richard-Devantoy S, Jollant F, Kefi Z, Turecki G, Olie JP, Annweiler C, et al: Deficit of cognitive inhibition in depressed elderly: a neurocognitive marker of suicidal risk. J Affect Disord 2012;140:193–199.
64 Richard-Devantoy S, Szanto K, Butters MA, Kalkus J, Dombrovski AY: Cognitive inhibition in older high-lethality suicide attempters. Int J Geriatr Psychiatry 2015;30:274–283.
65 Dombrovski AY, Szanto K, Siegle GJ, Wallace ML, Forman SD, Sahakian B, et al: Lethal forethought: delayed reward discounting differentiates high- and low-lethality suicide attempts in old age. Biol Psychiatry 2011;70:138–144.
66 McGirr A, Dombrovski AY, Butters MA, Clark L, Szanto K: Deterministic learning and attempted suicide among older depressed individuals: cognitive assessment using the Wisconsin card sorting task. J Psychiatr Res 2012;46:226–232.
67 Keilp JG, Gorlyn M, Russell M, Oquendo MA, Burke AK, Harkavy-Friedman J, et al: Neuropsychological function and suicidal behavior: attention control, memory and executive dysfunction in suicide attempt. Psychol Med 2013;43:539–551.
68 Swann AC, Dougherty DM, Pazzaglia PJ, Pham M, Steinberg JL, Moeller FG: Increased impulsivity associated with severity of suicide attempt history in patients with bipolar disorder. Am J Psychiatry 2005;162:1680–1687.
69 Dougherty DM, Mathias CW, Marsh DM, Papageorgiou TD, Swann AC, Moeller FG: Laboratory measured behavioral impulsivity relates to suicide attempt history. Suicide Life Threat Behav 2004;34:374–385.
70 Pettersen K, Rydningen NN, Christensen TB, Walby FA: Autobiographical memory and suicide attempts in schizophrenia. Suicide Life Threat Behav 2010;40:369–375.
71 Arie M, Apter A, Orbach I, Yefet Y, Zalzman G: Autobiographical memory, interpersonal problem solving, and suicidal behavior in adolescent inpatients. Compr Psychiatry 2008;49:22–29.
72 Kaviani H, Rahimi-Darabad P, Naghavi HR: Autobiographical memory retrieval and problem-solving deficits of Iranian depressed patients attempting suicide. J Psychopathol Behav Assess 2005;27:39–44.
73 Pollock LR, Williams JM: Problem-solving in suicide attempters. Psychol Med 2004;34:163–167.
74 Williams JM, Ellis NC, Tyers C, Healy H, Rose G, MacLeod AK: The specificity of autobiographical memory and imageability of the future. Mem Cognit 1996;24:116–125.
75 Williams JM, Broadbent K: Autobiographical memory in suicide attempters. J Abnorm Psychol 1986;95:144–149.
76 Maurex L, Lekander M, Nilsonne A, Andersson EE, Asberg M, Ohman A: Social problem solving, autobiographical memory, trauma, and depression in women with borderline personality disorder and a history of suicide attempts. Br J Clin Psychol 2010;49:327–342.
77 Taylor PJ, Gooding PA, Wood AM, Tarrier N: Memory specificity as a risk factor for suicidality in non-affective psychosis: the ability to recall specific autobiographical memories is related to greater suicidality. Behav Res Ther 2010;48:1047–1052.
78 Williams JM, Barnhofer T, Crane C, Beck AT: Problem solving deteriorates following mood challenge in formerly depressed patients with a history of suicidal ideation. J Abnorm Psychol 2005;114:421–431.
79 Crane C, Duggan DS: Overgeneral autobiographical memory and age of onset of childhood sexual abuse in patients with recurrent suicidal behaviour. Br J Clin Psychol 2009;48:93–100.
80 Rasmussen SA, O'Connor RC, Brodie D: The role of perfectionism and autobiographical memory in a sample of parasuicide patients: an exploratory study. Crisis 2008;29:64–72.

81 Sinclair JM, Crane C, Hawton K, Williams JM: The role of autobiographical memory specificity in deliberate self-harm: correlates and consequences. J Affect Disord 2007;102:11–18.
82 Startup M, Heard H, Swales M, Jones B, Williams JM, Jones RS: Autobiographical memory and parasuicide in borderline personality disorder. Br J Clin Psychol 2001;40:113–120.
83 Keilp JG, Gorlyn M, Russell M, Oquendo MA, Burke AK, Harkavy-Friedman J, et al: Neuropsychological function and suicidal behavior: attention control, memory and executive dysfunction in suicide attempt. Psychol Med 2013;43:539–551.
84 Jollant F, Guillaume S, Jaussent I, Bechara A, Courtet P: When knowing what to do is not sufficient to make good decisions: deficient use of explicit understanding in remitted patients with histories of suicidal acts. Psychiatry Res 2013;210:485–490.
85 Richard-Devantoy S, Jollant F, Kefi Z, Turecki G, Olie JP, Annweiler C, et al: Deficit of cognitive inhibition in depressed elderly: a neurocognitive marker of suicidal risk. J Affect Disord 2012;140:193–199.
86 Raust A, Slama F, Mathieu F, Roy I, Chenu A, Koncke D, et al: Prefrontal cortex dysfunction in patients with suicidal behavior. Psychol Med 2007;37:411–419.
87 Kim C, Jayathilake K, Meltzer F: Hopelessness, neurocognitive function, and insight in schizophrenia: a relationship to suicidal behavior. Schizophr Res 2003;60:71–80.
88 Nangle JM, Clarke S, Morris DW, Schwaiger S, McGhee KA, Kenny N, et al: Neurocognition and suicidal behaviour in an Irish population with major psychotic disorders. Schizophr Res 2006;85:196–200.
89 Keilp JG, Sackeim HA, Brodsky BS, Oquendo MA, Malone KM, Mann JJ: Neuropsychological dysfunction in depressed suicide attempters. Am J Psychiatry 2001;158:735–741.
90 Keilp JG, Wyatt G, Gorlyn M, Oquendo MA, Burke AK, John Mann J: Intact alternation performance in high lethality suicide attempters. Psychiatry Res 2014;219:129–136.
91 Potkin SG, Anand R, Alphs L, Fleming K: Neurocognitive performance does not correlate with suicidality in schizophrenic and schizoaffective patients at risk for suicide. Schizophr Res 2003;59:59–66.
92 Mann JJ: Neurobiology of suicidal behaviour. Nat Rev Neurosci 2003;4:819–828.
93 Turecki G, Ernst C, Jollant F, Labonte B, Mechawar N: The neurodevelopmental origins of suicidal behavior. Trends Neurosci 2012;35:14–23.
94 McGirr A, Turecki G: The relationship of impulsive aggressiveness to suicidality and other depression-linked behaviors. Curr Psychiatry Rep 2007;9:460–466.
95 Szanto K, Reynolds CF 3rd, Conwell Y, Begley AE, Houck P: High levels of hopelessness persist in geriatric patients with remitted depression and a history of attempted suicide. J Am Geriatr Soc 1998;46:1401–1406.
96 Beck AT, Steer RA, Kovacs M, Garrison B: Hopelessness and eventual suicide: a 10-year prospective study of patients hospitalized with suicidal ideation. Am J Psychiatry 1985;142:559–563.
97 Abrahams N, Jewkes R, Martin LJ, Mathews S, Vetten L, Lombard C: Mortality of women from intimate partner violence in South Africa: a national epidemiological study. Violence Vict 2009;24:546–556.
98 Keilp JG, Beers SR, Burke AK, Melhem NM, Oquendo MA, Brent DA, et al: Neuropsychological deficits in past suicide attempters with varying levels of depression severity. Psychol Med 2014;44:2965–2974.
99 Barrett EA, Sundet K, Simonsen C, Agartz I, Lorentzen S, Mehlum L, et al: Neurocognitive functioning and suicidality in schizophrenia spectrum disorders. Compr Psychiatry 2011;52:156–163.
100 Delaney C, McGrane J, Cummings E, Morris DW, Tropea D, Gill M, et al: Preserved cognitive function is associated with suicidal ideation and single suicide attempts in schizophrenia. Schizophr Res 2012;140:232–236.
101 Olie E, Seyller M, Beziat S, Loftus J, Bellivier F, Bougerol T, et al: Clinical and neuropsychological characteristics of euthymic bipolar patients having a history of severe suicide attempt. Acta Psychiatr Scand 2015;131:129–138.
102 Lopez-Castroman J, Courtet P, Baca-Garcia E, Oquendo MA: Identification of suicide risk in bipolar disorder. Bipolar Disord 2015;17:22–23.
103 Oquendo MA, Placidi GP, Malone KM, Campbell C, Keilp J, Brodsky B, et al: Positron emission tomography of regional brain metabolic responses to a serotonergic challenge and lethality of suicide attempts in major depression. Arch Gen Psychiatry 2003;60:14–22.
104 Gujral S, Dombrovski AY, Butters M, Clark L, Reynolds CF 3rd, Szanto K: Impaired executive function in contemplated and attempted suicide in late life. Am J Geriatr Psychiatry 2013, Epub ahead of print.
105 Walton ME, Behrens TE, Buckley MJ, Rudebeck PH, Rushworth MF: Separable learning systems in the macaque brain and the role of orbitofrontal cortex in contingent learning. Neuron 2010;65:927–939.
106 Dombrovski AY, Szanto K, Clark L, Aizenstein HJ, Chase HW, Reynolds CF, et al: Corticostriatothalamic reward prediction error signals and executive control in late-life depression. Psychol Med 2015;45:1413–1424.

107 Alichniewicz KK, Brunner F, Klunemann HH, Greenlee MW: Neural correlates of saccadic inhibition in healthy elderly and patients with amnestic mild cognitive impairment. Front Psychol 2013;4: 467.

108 Harrison BJ, Shaw M, Yucel M, Purcell R, Brewer WJ, Strother SC, et al: Functional connectivity during Stroop task performance. Neuroimage 2005;24: 181–191.

109 Coderre EL, van Heuven WJ: Modulations of the executive control network by stimulus onset asynchrony in a Stroop task. BMC Neurosci 2013;14:79.

110 Milham MP, Erickson KI, Banich MT, Kramer AF, Webb A, Wszalek T, et al: Attentional control in the aging brain: insights from an fMRI study of the Stroop task. Brain Cogn 2002;49:277–296.

111 Kane MJ, Engle RW: The role of prefrontal cortex in working-memory capacity, executive attention, and general fluid intelligence: an individual-differences perspective. Psychon Bull Rev 2002;9:637–671.

112 McDowd JM, Oseas-Kreger DM, Filion DL: Inhibitory processes in cognition and aging; in Dempster FN, Brainerd CJ (eds): Interference and Inhibition in Cognition. San Diego, Academic Press, 1995, pp 363–397.

113 Sublette ME, Milak MS, Galfalvy HC, Oquendo MA, Malone KM, Mann JJ: Regional brain glucose uptake distinguishes suicide attempters from non-attempters in major depression. Arch Suicide Res 2013;17:434–447.

114 Noonan MP, Walton ME, Behrens TE, Sallet J, Buckley MJ, Rushworth MF: Separate value comparison and learning mechanisms in macaque medial and lateral orbitofrontal cortex. Proc Natl Acad Sci U S A 2010;107:20547–20552.

115 Glascher J, Adolphs R, Damasio H, Bechara A, Rudrauf D, Calamia M, et al: Lesion mapping of cognitive control and value-based decision making in the prefrontal cortex. Proc Natl Acad Sci U S A 2012; 109:14681–14686.

116 Dombrovski AY, Szanto K, Clark L, Reynolds CF, Siegle GJ: Reward signals, attempted suicide, and impulsivity in late-life depression. JAMA Psychiatry 2013, Epub ahead of print.

Philippe Courtet, MD, PhD
Department of Emergency Psychiatry and Post-Acute Care, Hospital Lapeyronie
Avenue Gaston Giraud
FR–34295 Montpellier Cedex 5 (France)
E-Mail philippe.courtet@univ-montp1.fr

Kaschka WP, Rujescu D (eds): Biological Aspects of Suicidal Behavior.
Adv Biol Psychiatry. Basel, Karger, 2016, vol 30, pp 101–109 (DOI: 10.1159/000434743)

Electroencephalographic Risk Markers of Suicidal Behaviour

Steve Hodgkinson[a] · Jürgen Steyer[a] · Wolfgang P. Kaschka[a] · Martin Jandl[b]

[a] Klinik für Psychiatrie und Psychotherapie I, Universitätsklinikum Ulm, ZfP Südwürttemberg, Ulm/Ravensburg, Germany; [b] Universitätsklinik für Psychiatrie und Psychotherapie Bern, Bern, Switzerland

Abstract

Since its inception nearly 100 years ago, EEG (electroencephalography) has offered a non-invasive approach to recording the intrinsic electrical activity of the brain. Despite its limitations and the advent of brain imaging techniques with superior spatial resolution, the millisecond temporal resolution of EEG makes it a valuable diagnostic tool in many clinical disciplines, including psychiatry. In this chapter, we review its use in the assessment of suicide risk in psychiatric patients. After a general introduction to the technique itself, the first section considers the findings from numerous studies that have investigated paroxysmal EEG dysrhythmias such as small sharp spikes and other abnormal sleep parameters (rapid-eye movement latency and duration) in relation to suicidal behaviour. We then outline why changes in EEG patterns in response to a range of aural and visual stimuli (event-related potentials) might offer the most robust means of detecting facets of personality such as impulsiveness/aggressiveness that often underpin suicidal behaviour. Finally, we look at the wider aspects of using EEG data as a predictor of suicidal behaviour and why this is problematic at the moment. In the chapter summary, we draw together the findings into these three areas of EEG research and consider whether there is a case for extending the use of EEG as a routine adjunct to other diagnostic approaches for identifying suicidal behaviour in psychiatric patients close to release from inpatient care.

One could imagine that the German neurologist Hans Berger immediately appreciated the potential of his discovery when, in 1924, he recorded the first rhythmical electrical activity emanating from a human brain – almost 50 years after Richard Caton had conducted his preliminary experiments on rat brains [1, 2]. These two pioneers of EEG (electroencephalography) have all but been forgotten but their work laid the foundations for what was, in its heyday, an extremely influential experimental approach in neuropsychiatry. Today, almost 100 years later, EEG continues to be used widely in clinical research but has been somewhat overshadowed by newer innovations such as fMRI (functional magnetic resonance imaging) [3] and MEG (magnetoencephalography) [4].

The biophysical principles of EEG are relatively simple. Electrodes are attached at one end to the scalp of a subject according to an internationally agreed coordinate system and at the other to one of the inputs of a differential amplifier. A reference voltage electrode (attached to the ear) runs to the second input of the differential amplifier. Weak electrical activity emanating from the outer layers of the brain passes through the skull and is detected by the scalp electrodes. The difference between the voltage from the scalp electrode and that of the reference electrode is amplified, digitized and displayed as a time-resolved trace.

However, the electrical activity detected by the scalp electrodes is an average of many thousands of neurons, making it difficult to ascertain the spatial location of any emergent pattern (an example of the 'inverse problem'). The effects of distance from source, intervening cerebrospinal fluid and the skull itself further degrade the spatial coordinates of any pattern. Accepting this as a considerable limitation for the study of electrical activity in specific brain regions, EEG also offers some considerable advantages over its younger competitors. The temporal resolution of an EEG signal is in the order of a few milliseconds and the EEG measures *actual* brain electrical activity, both of which cannot be matched by fMRI or techniques such as SPECT (single photon emission computed tomography) which are much slower (several seconds or more) and measure changes in blood flow (an indirect measure of brain activity).

Normal brain activity measured using EEG may be conveniently divided into transient and rhythmic activity, the latter of which is classified by frequency. Of the six rhythmic frequency 'bands'; alpha (α), beta (β), gamma (γ), delta (δ), theta (θ) and mu (μ), only alpha wave patterns (7–14 Hz) have really been explored in relation to suicidal behaviour.

Graae et al. [5] recorded EEGs from a group of female Hispanic suicide attempters (n = 16) and controls (n = 22) and found that alpha wave asymmetry, whereby normally one observes greater right-side versus left-side alpha wave activity (less activation), was reversed in the suicidal behaviour group compared to the control group. Interestingly, Graae et al. reported a difference between depressed (n = 9) and non-depressed (n = 5) suicide attempters in terms of reversed alpha asymmetry. In the non-depressed suicide attempter group this was predominantly in the posterior region of the left hemisphere, whilst for the depressed suicide attempter group this was predominantly in the anterior region of the left hemisphere. Thus, whilst caution is needed when drawing conclusions from such small samples, reversed alpha asymmetry (reduced left posterior activation) may be more a marker for suicidal behaviour *per se* than for suicidal behaviour stemming from depressive illness.

Abnormal EEG Recordings during Sleep

Perhaps not surprisingly, given the complexity and susceptibility to external stimuli of the EEG source signal, attempts have been made to identify differences in the relatively well-defined phases of EEG activity occurring whilst the patient is asleep. Two main phases of sleep can be identified, non-rapid eye movement (NREM) and rapid eye movement (REM). On the basis of changes in EEG patterns, NREM may be further divided into stages I, II, III, and IV. In the first stages of NREM (I/II), alpha activity gradually decreases and becomes fragmented, giving way to so-called 'sleep spindles' and K complexes. During this period, theta activity increases. Stages II and IV are commonly known as slow-wave/delta sleep and representative EEG activity is only captured by extended (24-hour) recordings.

Due to the latency of REM sleep (around 100 min after stage I sleep), EEG activity during sleep is normally only captured by extended polysomnographic recordings. Longer recording identify distinctive EEG waveforms. REM sleep is characterized by EEG desynchronization, whereby faster, lower amplitude beta and theta activity replace the slow-wave sleep observed during stages II and IV of NREM.

Characterization of EEG patterns during sleep in patients exhibiting suicidal behaviour has focused mainly on the later stages of NREM or on the REM period of sleep. Some consistent findings have emerged. In the run-up to REM sleep, during stage IV of NREM, delta activity appears to be shorter in patients with depression who also present with suicidal behaviour compared to patients with depression who do not. This is mirrored by the general finding that latency to REM sleep is diminished in the former group when compared to data from non-suicidal depressed patients. In addition, REM time itself appears generally to be longer in those exhibiting suicidal behaviour [6–8]. However, in the absence of a plausible link between disturbed sleep patterns and the onset of suicidal behaviour, such observations have limited explanatory power. That link may well be a dysfunction of the serotonergic regulatory system.

Given the long-standing association between suicidal behaviour and dysfunctional serotonergic transmission [9], the latter also being intimately tied to the regulation of sleep patterns [10], it is tempting to speculate (as others have already done) that changes in serotonin production [11, 12], release [13] and, perhaps more controversially, reuptake[14] consistently found in patients with depression and suicidal behaviour may lead to a loss of regulatory control of the emotion centre found in the temporal lobes of the brain, the amygdala [15, 16].

Paroxysmal EEG Events: Small Sharp Spikes

During the first two stages of NREM sleep, sporadic, rapid spikes of activity known as small sharp spikes (SSS) occur. These spikes of activity (~50 mV) normally last for <50 ms and are broadly distributed across the temporal region of the brain [17]. In a series of studies, Struve et al. [17, 18] recorded paroxysmal EEG events (including SSS) in patients with a history of suicide attempts, together with a non-suicide attempt control group. They found a significant association between the presence of SSS and suicidal ideation/attempts. However, a later study of non-psychiatric patients and control subjects, the latter deprived of sleep for 24 h, suggests that SSS appear to be present in about 20% of individuals in *both* groups [19]. A study by Volow et al. [20] muddied the waters further by finding an increased incidence of paroxysmal events in the EEGs of patients with a history of suicidal behaviour (14.9%) compared to a group with no history of suicidal behaviour (6.6%) but this was not statistically significant. Thus, although Struve et al. [17, 18] found that all of the patients exhibiting suicidal behaviour also had SSS, the significant degree of overlap between suicidal and non-suicidal groups makes the use of SSS problematic without further refinement of the clinico-psychological features of suicidal behaviour and a more detailed analysis of SSS patterns.

EEG Event-Related Potentials

The inter-subject variability and general complexity of the EEG present a formidable barrier to its use as a means of distinguishing one group of subjects from another. Thus, the possibility of capturing so-called 'time-locked' EEG activity where changes in the EEG of an individual can be linked to some specific stimulus is appealing. Such changes in the EEG trace are called event-related potentials (ERPs) and were first described by Davis et al. [21] over 75 years ago. ERPs are classified according to their post-stimulus latency as either exogenous (sensory) or endogenous (cognitive). Fast exogenous ERPs occur <100 ms after the stimulus and represent a direct (precognitive) sensory response to the stimulus, whereas the slower endogenous ERPs take longer to appear as they also reflect the time taken to evaluate sensory data.

A commonly reported auditory-evoked positive potential occurring 50 ms after the stimulus (hence P50) is thought to identify a sensory gating mechanism whereby non-salient sensory information is filtered out. Two paradigms are frequently employed for investigating the P50 auditory-evoked response. The first involves generating a series (at intervals of 10 s) of pairs of audible clicks (500 ms apart). In control subjects, the second ERP is normally attenuated with respect to the first. The second approach, called mismatch negativity, involves interrupting the normal pattern of two 'standard' stimuli with a 'deviant' stimulus. In control subjects this deviant stimulus elicits a well-documented negative peak on the EEG which is much greater than the negative peak of the (attenuated) auditory ERP generated by the standard stimulus. The sensory gating of auditory-evoked P50 ERPs has been shown to be abnormal in a number of psychiatric disorders, most notably in schizophrenia [22].

P50 and P200 gating latency abnormalities have also been observed in patients with bipolar I disorder [23]. However, although just over half of the patients with bipolar I disorder had a history of suicidal ideation or attempts, no specific association was reported between suicidal ideation/attempts and P50/P200 gating irregularities.

By contrast, irregularities in the P300 ERP pattern have been found in a range of psychiatric disorders, including schizophrenia [24] and bipolar disorder [25]. In fact, the robustness of the P300 ERP to discriminate between patient and control groups in a range of more general studies probably explains why P300 irregularities have also been reported by a small number of groups specifically interested in its potential as a marker for suicidal behaviour [26–28]. What emerges from these studies is a mixed picture. The two earlier studies compared P300 amplitudes in patients with bipolar I disorder versus controls, with one study (Hansenne et al. [26], 1996) finding a negative correlation between P300 amplitude (measured at the central, midline electrode; Cz) and suicide attempts and the other (Chen et al. [27], 2005) finding a positive correlation. In a more recent study, Jandl et al. [28] (2009) compared P300 habituation in patients with major depressive disorder grouped according to whether they had no history of suicidal behaviour or had made 'soft' (poisoning) or 'hard' (jumping from a high object, hanging, stabbing) attempts at suicide. An extended 'oddball' paradigm was employed, where three stimuli (target/non-target and novel non-target) were delivered with differing probability, e.g. target 650 Hz (10%)/non-target 500 Hz (80%)/ novel different environmental sounds (10%), and the subject was required to discriminate the infrequent target stimulus from the more frequent non-target stimulus by noting the occurrence of the target by pressing a button.

Jandl et al. [28] found a quicker P300 habituation to both target and novel stimuli in patients with major depressive disorder *and* a history of suicidal behaviour compared to those who did not. Interestingly, all three of the studies mentioned above indicate that the changes in P300 activity observed in patients with affective disorder and a history of suicidal behaviour are only associated with their suicidality and not with the severity of their depressive illness.

The P300 ERP is essentially an electrophysiological marker for an informative external event or stimulus and as such probably reflects the processing/summation of neural signals into the consciousness. As such, the amplitude of the P300 ERP can reflect (depending on the task design) how unusual or unexpected a stimulus is or (not surprisingly) the degree of motivation and vigilance exhibited by the subject [29]. The P300 response is now known to consist of (at least) two components, the so-called P3a and P3b [30]. P3a is recorded predominantly in the frontal regions and is elicited by novel stimuli interspersed within a series of regular stimuli. P3a identifies a 'what is it?' orienting response to novel stimuli but exhibits relatively rapid habituation. By contrast, the P3b response is recorded in the parietal regions of the brain and occurs in situations where a subject makes a physical movement such as pressing a button in response to a novel stimulus.

As such the P300 is a 'man for all seasons' marker which is at once useful, as it enables many different aspects of cognitive processing in patients with mental illness to be investigated, but also perplexing as its complexity makes it more difficult to ascertain what actually is going on within the brains of patients that is so different to that of their non-patient counterparts.

A brief diversion back into the work of Ray Johnson Jr. is useful at this stage. Johnson outlined a taxonomy of factors that are reflected in P300 amplitude [31]. Three underlying dimensions were identified – subjective probability, stimulus meaning and information transmission – the former two having independent, additive effects on P300 amplitude, whilst the latter, information transmission, acts as a modulator. Thus, subjective probability captures the a priori likelihood of an event as judged by the test subject. The stimulus meaning refers to the task/stimulus complexity and the stimulus value. Finally, the information transmission dimension depicts the proportion of the stimulus/task information the test subject attends to.

Why is all of this important for assessing the data that has emerged from studies of P300 amplitude in patients with suicidal behaviour? Nearly 40 years ago, Shiffrin and Schneider [32] proposed two forms of cognitive operations, so-called automatic and controlled processing. Automatic processing functions continuously and is not modulated by the intent of the individual, whilst controlled processing *is* dependent upon the intent of the individual. Considerable data exists to suggest that automatic processing is responsible for the subjective probability dimension of Johnson [31], whilst controlled processing has a primary role in the stimulus meaning dimension [33]. Lower P300 amplitude and faster P300 habituation found in patients with a history of suicidal behaviour appear not to be attributable to the severity of depression or schizophrenia but rather to the presence (and possible severity) of suicidal behaviour itself. Hence, in such patients, the presence of suicidal behaviour should be associated with changes in either automatic or controlled processing or both. The standard paradigms (e.g. oddball) currently employed are not able to resolve the relative contributions of automatic and controlled processing to the lowering of the P300 amplitude or to its faster habituation. Such fine resolution may only be achieved by paradigms that employ multiple stimuli with different patterns (automatic processing) and that vary the task complexity (controlled processing).

A Predictive Role for EEG in Suicide Prevention?

One example of where a more finely resolved EEG investigation might be particularly useful is in the elucidation of the role of impulsivity in suicidal behaviour [34]. There is an ongoing debate regarding the extent to which the act of committing suicide is premeditated or impulsive. Its consideration now extends beyond the clinical aspects of suicidal behaviour to encompass the personal liability of individuals and the corporate liability of organization when a patient commits suicide [35]. Here the question of impulsivity becomes paramount as it delineates the 'impulsive' act of suicide as being (largely) unforeseeable. There is a danger that a failure to detect any suicidal intent during a pre-discharge interview will always be explained by the impulsive nature of the subsequent suicide [36]. Thus, a much better understanding of the *background* role of impulsivity within the constellation of factors that transform suicidal intent into the act of committing suicide is needed. For example, Joiner [37] has proposed that impulsivity should be conceptualized as a personality trait whereby certain individuals engage in risk-taking behaviour, which over time establishes the capability in some (not all) to enact serious harm to themselves. Viewed this way, impulsivity is not enough to predict suicidal behaviour; rather it predicts the capability to commit suicide if there are also well-defined plans to do so.

Viewed from this perspective, the use of EEG as one of a battery of procedures to screen for trait impulsivity in admitted patients alongside detailed observations and notes regarding suicidal plans and intentions would seem prudent. This would remove the problem of elevating the role of EEG to be the predictor of suicidal behaviour which it clearly cannot fill.

Conclusion

It is easy to believe that EEG will play an ever-decreasing role in the elucidation of how the observed disturbances in brain activity found in patients with a mental illness reflect the symptoms they describe. The advent of highly sophisticated and spatially defined approaches to recording the electrophysiological activity of the brain cast a substantial shadow over the technique that Berger [1] introduced to the world nearly a century ago. However, interest in EEG endures, partly because of its simplicity and immediacy but also because it has produced some very robust results over the years about how the brain responds to a range of stimuli. Much of the potential of EEG remains untapped as the repertoire of paradigms used for its deployment remains small. The use of paradigms that explore some of the ideas outlined in the model of Johnson [31] might be a good start, allowing a much better assessment to be made of the possible association between suicidal behaviour and impulsivity.

The raison d'être for much of the work attempting to find specific (anomalous) patterns of EEG activity in depressed patients that also exhibit suicidal behaviour is the possibility of establishing a definitive set of correlates that are predictive of such behaviour in general and are therefore useful as a diagnostic marker. Given that a significant number of patients with a depressive illness who commit suicide subsequent to their release from hospital report no suicidal behaviour [38], such a marker would indeed be very useful.

References

1 Berger H: Über das Elektrenkephalogramm des Menschen. Archiv f. Psychiatrie u. Nervenkrankheiten 1929;87:527–570.

2 Ogawa S, Lee TM, Kay AR, Tank DW: Brain magnetic resonance imaging with contrast dependent upon blood oxygenation. Proc Natl Acad Sci 1990; 87:9868–9872.

3 Caton R: The electric currents of the brain. Brit Med J 1875;2:278.

4 Cohen D: Magnetoencephalography: detection of the brain's electrical activity with a superconducting magnetometer. Science 1972;175:664–666.

5 Graae F, Tenke G, Bruder G, RotheramM-J, Piacentini J, Castro-Blanco D, Leite P, Towey J: Abnormality of EEG alpha asymmetry in female adolescent suicide attempters. Biol Psychiatry 1996;40:706–713.

6 Sabo E, Reynolds CF 3rd, Kupfer DJ, Berman SR: Sleep, depression and suicide. Psychiatry Res 1991; 36:265–277.

7 Dahl RE, Puig-Antich J, Ryan ND, Nelson B, Dachille S, Cunningham SL, Trubnick L, Klepper TP: EEG sleep in adolescents with major depression: the role of suicidality and inpatient status. J Affect Disord 1990;19:63–75.

8 Agargun MY, Cartwright R: REM sleep, dream variables and suicidality in depressed patients. Psychiatry Res 2003;119:33–39.

9 Van Heeringen C: Suicide, serotonin and the brain. Crisis 2001;22:66–70.

10 Jouvet M: Sleep and serotonin: an unfinished story. Neuropsychopharmacology 1999;21(2 suppl):24S–27S.

11 Åsberg M, Träskman L, Thorén P: 5-HIAA in the cerebrospinal fluid: a biochemical suicide predictor? Arch Gen Psychiatry 1976;33:1193–1197.

12 Mann JJ: Neurobiology of suicidal behaviour. Nat Rev Neurosci 2003;4:819–828.

13 Oquendo MA, Placidi GP, Malone KM, Campbell C, Keilp J, Brodsky B, Kegeles LS, Cooper TB, Parsey RV, Van Heertum RL, Mann JJ: Positron emission tomography for regional brain metabolic responses to a serotonergic challenge and lethality of suicide attempts in major depression. Arch Gen Psychiatry 2003;60:14–22.

14 Björkenstam C, Möller J, Ringbäck G, Salmi P, Hallqvist J, Ljung R: An association between initiation of selective serotonin reuptake inhibitors and suicide – a nationwide register-based case-crossover study. PLoS One 2013;8:e73973.

15 Tran L, Lasher BK, Young KA, Keele NB: Depletion of serotonin in the basolateral amygdale elevates glutamate receptors and facilitates fear-potentiated startle. Transl Psychiatry 2013;3:e298.

16 Volman I, Verhagen L, den Ouden HE, Fernández G, Rijpkema M, Franke B, Toni I, Roelofs K: Reduced serotonin transporter availability decreases prefrontal control of the amygdala. J Neurosci 2013;33: 8974–8979.

17 Struve FA, Klein DF, Saraf KR: Electroencephalographic correlates of suicide ideation and attempts. Arch Gen Psychiatry 1972;27:363–365.

18 Struve FA, Saraf KR, Arko RS, Klein DF, Becker DR: Relationship between paroxysmal electroencephalographic dysrhythmia and suicide ideation and attempts in psychiatric patients; in Shagass C, Gershon S, Friedhoff AJ (eds): Psychopathology and Brain Dysfunction. New York, Raven Press, pp 199–221.

19 White JC, Langston JW, Pedley TA: Benign epileptiform transients of sleep. Clarification of the small sharp spike controversy. Neurology 1997;27:1061–1068.

20 Volow MR, Zung WW, Green RL: Electroencephalographic abnormalities in suicidal patients. J Clin Psychiatry 1979;40:213–216.

21 Davis H, Davis PA, Loomis AL, Harvey EN, Hobart G: Electrical reactions of the human brain to auditory stimulation during sleep. J Neurophysiol 1939; 2:500–514.

22 Freedman R, Adler LE, Gerhardt GA, Waldo M, Baker N, Rose GM, Drebing C, Nagamoto H, Bickford-Wimmer P, Franks R: Neurobiological studies of sensory gating in schizophrenia. Schizophr Bull 1987;13:669–677.

23 Lijffijt M, Moeller LG, Boutros NN, Steinberg JL, Meier SL, Lane SD, Swann AC: Diminished P50, n100 and P200 auditory sensory gating in bipolar I disorder. Psychiatry Res 2009;167:191–201.

24 Mathalon DH, Ford JM, Pfefferbaum A: Trait and state aspects of p300 amplitude reduction in schizophrenia: a retrospective longitudinal study. Biol Psychiatry 2000;47:434–449.

25 O'Donnell BF, Vohs JL, Hetrick WP, Carroll CA, Shekhar A: Auditory event-related potential abnormalities in bipolar disorder and schizophrenia. Int J Psychophysiology 2004;53:45–55.

26 Hansenne M, Pichot W, Gonzales Morino A, Zaldua IU, Ansseau M: Suicidal behavior in depressive disorder: an event-related potential study. Biol Psychiatry 1996;40:116–122.

27 Chen TJ, Yu YW, Chen MC, Wang SY, Tsai SJ, Lee TW: Serotonin dysfunction and suicide attempts in major depressives: an auditory event-related potential study. Neuropsychobiology 2005;52:28–36.

28 Jandl M, Steyer J, Kaschka WP: Suicide risk markers in major depressive disorder: a study of electrodermal activity and event-related potentials. J Affect Disord 2009;123:138–149.

29 Hansenne M: Event-related brain potentials in psychopathology: clinical and cognitive perspectives. Psychol Belg 2006;46:5–36.
30 Squires NK, Squires KC, Hillyard SA: Two varieties of long latency positive waves evoked by unpredictable auditory stimuli in man. Electroencephalogr Clin Neurophysiol 1975;38:387–401.
31 Johnson R Jr: A triarchic model of P300 amplitude. Psychophysiology 1986;23:67–84.
32 Shiffrin RM, Schneider W: Controlled and automatic human information processing. II. Perceptual learning, automatic attending, and a general theory. Psychol Rev 1977;84:127–190.
33 Hasher L, Zacks RT: Automatic processing of fundamental information: the case of frequency of occurrence. Am Psychol 1984;39:1372–1388.
34 Wyder M, De Leo D: Behind impulsive suicide attempts: indications from a community study. J Affect Disord 2007;104:167–173.
35 Smith AR, Witte TK, Teale NE, King SL, Bender TW, Joiner TE: Revisiting impulsivity in suicide: implications for civil liability of third parties. Behav Sci Law 2008;26:779–797.
36 Carey B: Making sense of the great suicide debate. New York Times, Week in Review, February 10, 2008.
37 Joiner TE: Why people die by suicide. Cambridge, Harvard University Press, 2005.
38 Dennehy J, Appleby L, Thomas C: Case-control study of suicide by discharged psychiatric patients. Br Med J 1996;312:1580.

Dr. Steve Hodgkinson
Klinik für Psychiatrie und Psychotherapie I, Universitätsklinikum Ulm, ZfP Südwürttemberg
Weingartshofer Strasse 2
DE–88214 Ravensburg (Germany)
E-Mail steve.hodgkinson@uni-ulm.de

Kaschka WP, Rujescu D (eds): Biological Aspects of Suicidal Behavior.
Adv Biol Psychiatry. Basel, Karger, 2016, vol 30, pp 110–122 (DOI: 10.1159/000434744)

Neuroimaging of Suicidal Behavior

Fabrice Jollant

Douglas Mental Health University Institute, McGill University, Montreal, Que., Canada; Academic Hospital (CHU) of Nîmes, Nîmes, France

Abstract

Over the last 15 years, an increasing number of studies have been conducted to investigate the neural basis of suicidal behavior in vivo, using neuroimaging. In this chapter, we will review the literature on the topic before proposing an updated version of our neurocognitive model. Review shows that few studies have used pharmacological neuroimaging to investigate brain receptors. Moreover, these studies present methodological issues including small sample size, thus limiting their interpretation. Spectroscopy has also been used too rarely to draw any firm conclusion so far. In contrast, structural neuroimaging has been extensively used and suggests reduced volumes, mainly in different parts of the prefrontal cortex, in addition to parietal and temporal cortices and possibly some subcortical nuclei. In addition, several studies have reported white matter lesions in individuals with histories of suicidal acts and mood disorders from adolescents to the elderly, suggesting impaired brain connectivity. Diffusion tensor imaging has not been used often to date but supports impaired connectivity, notably to the orbitofrontal cortex. Finally, functional neuroimaging studies have highlighted impaired responses in suicide attempters to various conditions, including decision making, social threat, cognitive control, verbal fluency, mental pain, and resting state. We propose that the vulnerability to suicidal behavior and the triggering of the suicidal crisis is related to a combination of trait and state deficits, including valuation processes on one side and cognitive control and self-referential processes on the other side. This would be underlain by a dysfunctional network of regions, including the ventral and dorsal parts of the prefrontal cortex and the parietal and temporal lobes. Future research should develop interventions targeting these neurocognitive alterations for the prevention of suicide.

Suicide and suicide attempts are complex human behaviors. As a consequence, explaining these behaviors will necessitate different methodological approaches, with the ultimate goal of combining the findings to form a general explicative model (or possibly models). Over the past decades, research on suicide has successfully applied new technologies to the study of suicidal acts, from genetics to epigenetics and cellular histology to biochemistry (see other chapters). Another expanding field of research at the interface of biology and clinical/psychological levels is neurocognition, which aims to integrate the study of the cognitive processes and their neuroanatomical basis.

The use of neuropsychological tasks in individuals with histories of suicidal acts dates back from the late 1960s but it was only in the early 2000s that robust protocols were implemented [1, 2]. Neuroimaging studies of suicidal behavior also started in the 2000s, using SPECT (single photon emission computed tomography) [3], PET (positron emission tomography) [4] and MRI (magnetic resonance imaging) [5]. These last 15 years have witnessed an increasing number of studies published with the goal of investigating the neurocognitive basis of suicidal acts.

I will focus in this chapter on neuroimaging findings, as neuropsychological results are presented elsewhere in this book, though both should be considered together for a comprehensive understanding of the suicidal mind. Before discussing the functional neuroimaging findings, we will discuss three other types of neuroimaging which focus primarily on the structure of the brain, namely pharmacological and structural neuroimaging and spectroscopy.

Pharmacological Neuroimaging

Pharmacological neuroimaging aims at exploring the binding of various ligands to particular receptors in vivo. As such, it allows for interesting bridges between biochemical systems, neuroanatomy and the vulnerability to suicidal acts. It therefore complements findings from both postmortem and in vivo studies, using peripheral measures in the cerebrospinal fluid or blood, for instance.

Not surprisingly, the serotonergic system has been the most studied. Cannon et al. [6], in secondary analyses of a study on bipolar disorder, reported reduced binding to the serotonin transporter (5-HTT) in the midbrain and increased binding in the anterior cingulate cortex of 8 unmedicated suicide attempters versus 10 patient controls. The same group [7] also reported increased 5-HTT binding in the anteroventral striatum in 6 attempters versus 12 patient controls with major depressive disorder and in the anterior cingulate cortex in 8 attempters versus 10 patient controls with bipolar disorder. Nye et al. [8] also found decreased binding in the midbrain of 11 unmedicated attempters versus 10 healthy controls. However, three other groups did not find any significant group difference in 5-HTT binding between 12 recent unmedicated suicide attempters and 12 healthy controls [9–11], 9 unmedicated attempters versus 9 patient controls with bipolar disorder [12] and 9 unmedicated suicide attempters and 16 patient controls with major depressive disorder [13].

The 5-HT_{2A} receptor has been investigated by three research groups. Audenaert et al. [3] found decreased binding in the frontal cortex of 12 individuals who recently committed a suicidal act versus 12 healthy controls, a measure that was correlated with harm avoidance and hopelessness [14]. Meyer et al. [15], in secondary analyses of a study on dysfunctional attitudes, found no binding difference between 18 patients with a history of self-harm and chronic suicidal ideation (mainly with borderline personality disorder) relative to 29 healthy controls, although binding was lower in those who committed a more severe suicidal act. Soloff et al. [16], in secondary analyses of a study on borderline personality disorder, reported increased binding in suicide attempters versus healthy controls in the hippocampus, medial temporal cortex and occipital cortex, with a trend in the lateral orbitofrontal cortex. These results were, however, very similar to those found in patients in general.

Finally, Leyton et al. [17] found reduced α-[^{11}C]methyl-L-tryptophan trapping, a marker of serotonin synthesis, in the orbital and ventromedial prefrontal cortex of 10 high-lethality suicide attempters versus 16 healthy controls. There was also a negative correlation between binding in the lateral orbitofrontal and medial prefrontal cortices and suicidal intent.

Outside the serotonergic system, only the dopamine transporter has been investigated by one research group, which found no binding difference between 12 attempters and 12 healthy controls [9–11].

Although pharmacological neuroimaging represents a potential valuable tool, this brief overview highlights the scarcity of studies using this technique, the limited interpretation of findings, mainly due to the small sample size of all studies (which were often secondary analyses), and the frequent lack of a patient control group to differentiate what is specifically related to suicidal acts from what is related to comorbid disorders like depression. More PET research using specifically designed studies is definitely needed.

Spectroscopy Neuroimaging

Spectroscopy uses MRI to measure the concentration of various biochemical compounds (including glutamate, GABA, N-acetyl-aspartate, myo-inositol…) in a localized part of the brain. One major drawback of this technique is the limited brain volume (actually a big voxel of $2.5 \times 2.5 \times 2.5$ cm^3, for instance) that can be assessed within one scanner session.

In the only published study using this technique in the context of suicidal behavior (a study published in Chinese), Li et al. [18] found reduced N-acetyl-aspartate/creatinine ratio in the left hippocampus of 24 suicide attempters versus 24 healthy controls and no patient control group. The results are more likely a reflection of a depressive state than the vulnerability to suicidal acts, as previously shown [19]. Again, more studies using this interesting technique are necessary.

Structural Neuroimaging

Lesion Studies

Since the early 2000s, several studies have reported an increased number of white matter signals (shown as hyperintensities in T2 MRI sequences) in suicide attempters versus patient controls. In elderly patients with unipolar depression, Ahearn et al. [5]

reported an increased number of subcortical gray matter hyperintensities and a trend for increased periventricular hyperintensities in attempters versus patient controls matched for age and gender. Sachs-Ericsson et al. [20] also found an increased number of white matter hyperintensities in 23 elderly suicide attempters versus 223 patient controls, with a greater growth of lesions in attempters over a 2-year follow-up period. In a large sample of 153 child and adolescent inpatients with various psychiatric diagnoses, Ehrlich et al. [21, 22] showed that white matter hyperintensities increased the risk of suicide attempts by 18 in patients with unipolar depression, notably deep white matter hyperintensities in the right parietal lobe. Similar results were found in 3 studies in middle-aged patients suffering from mood disorders, with more hyperintensities, specifically periventricular hyperintensities, in attempters versus patient controls [22–24]. White matter lesions are one of the most replicated findings in neuroimaging of suicidal behavior and are found across different age groups. Results have mainly been reported in depressive disorder.

Interpretation remains difficult. It is suggested that these lesions may interfere with important connections, possibly anteroposterior tracts, and lead to deficits in significant cognitive and emotional processes. However, more investigations of the anatomical-cognitive correlations would be necessary to validate this hypothesis. Also, it would be important to investigate other psychiatric populations outside unipolar depression.

Morphometric Differences

Numerous studies have examined morphometric differences in brain regions in suicide attempters relative to controls. Differences in volumes have mainly been examined and more rarely differences in cortical thickness. Unfortunately, studies differ in several aspects regarding the strength of the magnetic field (1.5 or 3 T), analysis technique (voxel or surface-based morphometry, whole brain vs. region-of-interest, ROI) or clinical population (mainly mood disorder, more rarely schizophrenia) making the direct comparison of results more complicated. As it would be too fastidious to detail each study, we will focus on brain regions.

Not surprisingly, if we consider previous postmortem studies [25], several morphometric differences have been reported in the prefrontal cortex. Findings support reduced volumes of various parts of this region, including the orbitofrontal and ventrolateral [26–28], medial and dorsomedial (including anterior cingulate cortex) [26, 29–32] and dorsolateral [26] prefrontal cortices. These results were found across various diagnoses, including mood disorders [26, 28, 30, 31], schizophrenia [27, 29] and borderline personality disorder [32], and across age groups including the elderly [31]. Opposite results are rarely reported. Rusch et al. [33] found increased white matter volumes in bilateral posterior orbital and inferior frontal gyri in patients with schizophrenia, with no difference in gray matter volume. Soloff et al. [34] found no volumetric differences in the prefrontal cortex of attempters with borderline personality disorder. However, reduced volume was found in high- versus low-lethality attempters in the orbitofrontal cortex in the same study. Finally, Wagner et al. [35] reported reduced thickness in the ventrolateral, dorsolateral and anterior cingulate cortices in a mixed group of patients at increased personal and familial suicide risk.

Apart from the prefrontal cortex, reduced cortical volumes were found in the insular [29, 31, 34], parietal [26, 29, 31], temporal [26, 27, 29, 31], and occipital [26, 29] lobes and the cerebellum [31]. Increased volumes were also reported, notably in the temporal cortex [26, 34]. An ROI approach showed no difference between attempters and nonattempters with bipolar disorder in cerebellar volume [36].

Subcortical nuclei have also been explored through whole-brain and sometimes ROI analyses. Reduced volumes in suicide attempters have been found in the thalamus [29], nucleus accumbens [29], basal ganglia [26], lentiform nucleus [31], putamen [37], caudate [38], and pallidum [38]. Dombrovski et al. [37] noted a significant association between higher delay discounting and lower putamen gray matter voxel counts. Lopez-Larson et al. [39] found increased thalamic volumes in a complex population of veterans with mild traumatic brain injury who attempted suicide. Dombrovski et al. [37] found no difference in caudate or putamen voxel counts. Two studies reported no difference in amygdala volumes in borderline personality disorder [34] and schizophrenia [27]. Spoletini et al. [40] found increased right amygdala volumes in attempters versus nonattempters with schizophrenia but no difference in the lateral ventricles, thalamus, hippocampus, caudate, putamen, pallidum, and accumbens. Monkul et al. [28] also reported increased amygdalar volume in a small sample of unmedicated female attempters versus nonattempters with unipolar depression. To our knowledge, the hippocampus has never been involved in the vulnerability to suicidal acts in any morphometric studies. As volumetric alterations have been related to histories of childhood abuse [41], hippocampus alterations may only apply to a subgroup of suicide attempters [42].

Other findings include a reduced posterior third of the corpus callosum in elderly patients [43], although this result was not replicated in another study in medicated patients with bipolar I disorder [44] and in another small sample [45]. Jovev et al. [46] found a positive correlation between pituitary gland volume and number of parasuicidal acts in borderline personality disorder in a study with no group comparison. Moreover, reduced volume of the midbrain has been reported in 1 study [31].

Finally, Benedetti et al. [26] showed that most reduced volumes found in suicide attempters were reversed by lithium, a drug with significant antisuicidal properties [47].

Diffusion Tensor Imaging

Diffusion tensor imaging (DTI) enables the indirect assessment of white matter morphology through the measure of the diffusion of water in tissues. Few studies on suicidal behavior have been published to date using this technique. Jia et al. [48, 49] reported reduced fractional anisotropy (the main DTI measure) in the left anterior limb of the internal capsule, which has projections to the thalamus and orbitofrontal cortex, and in the right lentiform nucleus in 16 suicide attempters versus 36 patient controls. Mahon et al. [50] reported lower fractional anisotropy in the left orbitofrontal white matter in 14 attempters versus 15 nonattempters with bipolar disorder. Olvet et al. [51] reported lower fractional anisotropy in the dorsomedial prefrontal cortex in 13 suicide attempters versus 39 patient controls. Lopez-Larson et al. [39] found increased fractional anisotropy in the thalamus in 19 attempters with mild traumatic brain injury.

Functional Neuroimaging

Decision Making and Reversal Learning

Impaired decision making has been associated with a history of suicidal behavior in a recent meta-analysis of 9 studies [52]. Jollant et al. [53] found that impaired decision making in 13 euthymic male middle-aged suicide attempters versus 12 patient controls was related to a decreased response of the left orbitofrontal cortex and occipital cortex to risky versus safe choices during the Iowa Gambling Task. Examination suggests that this region does not correctly encode the contrast between risky and safe choices in attempters, the magnitude of the difference being positively correlated with final performance. A replication study (Olié et al., submitted) confirmed decreased activation in the left ventrolateral, but also in the left dorsolateral, prefrontal cortex in 15 suicide attempters versus 23 patient controls. Moreover, preliminary analyses suggest that healthy first-degree relatives of suicide completers also show decision-making impairment and that these alterations are related to decreased activation of the ventromedial prefrontal cortex, with the same pattern of decreased activation contrast during risky and safe choices (article in preparation). Decision-making impairment may therefore be heritable and may be related to deficits in risk valuation processes in the ventral and perhaps dorsolateral prefrontal cortices.

Another study in adolescents has been conducted with the same task but results are difficult to interpret as many participants could not complete the task [54].

Dombrovski et al. [55] found reduced response to expected reward during a reversal learning task in the ventromedial prefrontal cortex in 15 elderly depressed suicide attempters versus 18 patient controls. This result is therefore close to those found with the decision-making task, with deficient valuation processing in the ventral prefrontal cortex in suicide attempters.

Cognitive and Motor Inhibition

In total, 3 studies have specifically investigated these cognitive processes in suicide attempters or completers. Cognitive control is a generic term that covers various processes, including cognitive inhibition, error detection, response conflict, and cognitive flexibility. In 2 articles (possibly overlapping sample), the authors have used HMPAO SPECT and the Conners continuous performance test to assess motor inhibition [56, 57]. The strength of this study is that the patients, unmedicated at the time of scanning, were followed after the initial assessment, with some ultimately committing suicide. In comparison to 12 noncompleters, the 12 completers showed increased activity at rest in an extensive area covering the right temporal, frontal, cingulate, parietal, insular, and occipital cortices, suggesting an excessive activation of the default mode network. During the task, completers had decreased activation in the frontal, medial temporal lobe and thalamus and increased activation in the anterior cingulate cortex, cerebellum and occipital lobe. In an extended sample, 21 completed suicides versus 27 heathy controls showed decreased activation during the task in the bilateral superior frontal lobes, right precuneus, rolandic operculum, postcentral gyrus, left caudate, insular cortex, and subgenual cingulate cortex.

In medicated depressed adolescent attempters, Pan et al. [58] reported decreased activation in the anterior cingulate cortex relative to patient controls during the go/no-go task.

Verbal Fluency

Verbal fluency abilities have been found deficient in attempters versus nonattempters [52]. Audenaert et al. [59], using SPECT, found decreased activation in 20 attempters versus 20 healthy controls in the inferior and middle frontal gyrus, inferior parietal gyrus and anterior cingulate cortex during category fluency and in the medial temporal gyrus, anterior cingulate cortex and hypothalamic region during letter fluency. The lack of a patient control group makes inferences complicated. In suicide attempters, Oquendo et al. [4] found brain activity in the anterior cingulate cortex and superior medial prefrontal cortex, measured at rest by PET, to be positively correlated with verbal fluency performance in suicide attempters.

Response to Angry Faces

Angry faces are signals of social threat, a relevant paradigm to test social stress in the context of suicidal acts. A first study in male normothymic middle-aged patients [60] showed an increased response of the right lateral orbitofrontal cortex to angry versus neutral faces, but not to happy faces, in 13 suicide attempters versus 14 patient controls. This result was recently replicated in another sample of male patients (Olié et al., submitted). Using the same task in depressed adolescents, Pan et al. [61] reported a different pattern of activation, with an increased response to subtle angry faces in 14 suicide attempters in the anterior cingulate, dorsolateral prefrontal, primary sensory, and temporal cortices. Sample bias and some specificities related to the immature brain may explain discrepancies between the 3 studies.

Mental Pain

Mental pain has been hypothesized to be central to the suicidal crisis [62]. A study in 10 female suicide attempters [63] used scripts describing the mental pain experienced just before the suicidal act and the act itself to evoke brain responses. The suicidal act script led to an increased response in the parahippocampal gyrus, cuneus, middle temporal gyrus, and cerebellum and a decreased response in the medial prefrontal cortex. Mental pain was associated with a decreased response in the medial prefrontal cortex, anterior cingulate cortex and hippocampus.

Resting State

A few studies investigated brain activity at rest, an activity associated with the default mode network, i.e. a network of regions activated when the individual is engaged in self-reflection or self-related tasks [64]. In a PET study, Oquendo et al. [4] found a decreased response in the anterior cingulate cortex and medial frontal gyrus in 16 high-lethality versus 9 low-lethality attempters – a contrast increased by a serotonergic probe. These measures were also correlated with suicidal intent and impulsivity. Using SPECT, Fountoulakis et al. [65] found no difference in brain activity between unmedicated depressed attempters and nonattempters. Fan et al. [66], using MRI, reported reduced activity in the ventromedial prefrontal cortex, parahippocampal gyrus, anterior cingulate cortex, and angular gyrus in 27 suicide attempters versus 10 patient controls but increased activity in the superior temporal gyrus. Finally, Sublette et al. [67] found decreased activity at rest in the dorsolateral prefrontal cortex in 13 suicide attempters versus 16 patient controls but increased activity in the ventromedial prefrontal cortex/orbitofrontal cortex, anterior cingulate, caudate, and putamen.

Conclusion

Taken together, the literature above suggests that the vulnerability to suicidal acts (as measured in patients with histories of suicide attempt relative to controls matched for comorbid disorders) is associated with several structural and functional brain abnormalities. Most differences have been found in the prefrontal cortex, including the ventral, medial and dorsolateral areas, in addition to the temporal and parietal cortices and possibly some subcortical nuclei. A recent meta-analysis of structural and functional neuroimaging studies [68] reported reduced volumes of the orbitofrontal cortex, superior temporal gyrus and caudate nucleus and increased reactivity of the anterior and posterior cingulate cortices. Furthermore, preliminary results suggest that some alterations may be heritable (article in preparation). Both white and gray matter alterations have been described, signifying complex regional and connectivity impairments. Another observation is that although most studies have been conducted in middle-aged patients, alterations have also been reported in adolescents and the elderly. However, direct comparisons across age groups have yet to be conducted. These findings could help disentangle the role of age in some neuroimaging findings. The same comment can be made for gender. Finally, most studies have been conducted in mood disorders, unipolar and bipolar disorders (both in euthymic and depressive states) and more rarely in schizophrenia. Some alterations seem to be found across these diagnoses, supporting the concept of transnosographic alterations specifically related to suicidal acts, even though some cognitive studies suggest different deficits in mood disorders and schizophrenia (with schizophrenic suicide attempters often showing better more than lower performance) [69].

A Tentative Neuroanatomical Model of Suicidal Behavior

We have previously presented an integrative working model of suicidal behavior at the neurocognitive level [70]. Here, we would like to propose an updated version of this model.

We believe that a central deficit in the vulnerability to suicidal acts is impaired valuation processes. This deficit is reflected in the following: (1) an increased response of the orbitofrontal cortex [60] and probably other prefrontal regions [61] to signals of social threat; (2) and to wins and versus losses in the prefrontal cortex (Olié et al., submitted); (3) but a lower response to expected reward in the ventromedial prefrontal cortex during reversal learning [55], and (4) risk during decision making in the orbitofrontal cortex and (probably dorsolateral) prefrontal cortex [53]. Another study showed an inability of suicide attempters to modulate response to unfairness [71]. Moreover, valuation deficit, largely related to the prefrontal cortex, would be a heritable trait (article in preparation). It would underlie persistent disadvantageous decision making, which is correlated with an increased risk of interpersonal relationship problems [72] – a classical trigger of suicidal crisis.

A second set of deficits is impaired cognitive control and self-related processing. Deficits in cognitive control are mainly associated with the mediodorsal prefrontal cortex [58], including the cingulate cortex and dorsolateral prefrontal cortex [73]. In combination with working memory deficits [74], they may limit the ability to regulate the emotional response in a stressful context, facilitating an obsessive and ruminative mode of thinking [75], mental pain [76], suicidal ideas [63], and intent [4]. Interestingly, we could not find any significant impairment in cognitive control in relatives of suicide completers who themselves never attempted suicide, suggesting that this may protect these individuals and counterbalance an otherwise decision-making impairment (article in preparation.). Moreover, the medial prefrontal cortex has also been associated with the default mode network and self-referential processes [64, 77] in connection with the temporal and parietal cortices. These self-related processes include autobiographical memory [64], which is found to be deficient in suicide attempters and correlated with deficient problem solving [74]. All these deficits could add to promote an inadequate perception of the self and future and limit the individual's abilities to find solutions to their problems [78], thus creating a feeling of hopelessness [78] and perhaps reducing help-seeking behavior.

In summary, deficits in valuation processes on one side and cognitive control and self-referential processes on the other side, mainly associated with dysfunctional prefrontal, parietal and temporal cortices, may represent the core neurocognitive basis of the vulnerability to suicidal acts. Interventions should be developed to target these deficits and assess their impact on the suicidal risk.

References

1 Keilp JG, Sackeim HA, Brodsky BS, Oquendo MA, Malone KM, Mann JJ: Neuropsychological dysfunction in depressed suicide attempters. Am J Psychiatry 2001;158:735–741.

2 Jollant F, Bellivier F, Leboyer M, et al: Impaired decision making in suicide attempters. Am J Psychiatry 2005;162:304–310.

3 Audenaert K, Van Laere K, Dumont F, et al: Decreased frontal serotonin 5-HT_{2A} receptor binding index in deliberate self-harm patients. Eur J Nucl Med 2001;28:175–182.

4 Oquendo MA, Placidi GP, Malone KM, et al: Positron emission tomography of regional brain metabolic responses to a serotonergic challenge and lethality of suicide attempts in major depression. Arch Gen Psychiatry 2003;60:14–22.

5 Ahearn EP, Jamison KR, Steffens DC, et al: MRI correlates of suicide attempt history in unipolar depression. Biol Psychiatry 2001;50:266–270.

6 Cannon DM, Ichise M, Fromm SJ, et al: Serotonin transporter binding in bipolar disorder assessed using [^{11}C]DASB and positron emission tomography. Biol Psychiatry 2006;60:207–217.

7 Cannon DM, Ichise M, Rollis D, et al: Elevated serotonin transporter binding in major depressive disorder assessed using positron emission tomography and [^{11}C]DASB; comparison with bipolar disorder. Biol Psychiatry 2007;62:870–877.

8 Nye JA, Purselle D, Plisson C, et al: Decreased brainstem and putamen SERT binding potential in depressed suicide attempters using [^{11}C]-ZIENT PET imaging. Depress Anxiety 2013;30:902–907.

9 Lindstrom MB, Ryding E, Bosson P, Ahnlide JA, Rosen I, Traskman-Bendz L: Impulsivity related to brain serotonin transporter binding capacity in suicide attempters. Eur Neuropsychopharmacol 2004;14:295–300.

10 Ryding E, Ahnlide JA, Lindstrom M, Rosen I, Traskman-Bendz L: Regional brain serotonin and dopamine transporter binding capacity in suicide attempters relate to impulsiveness and mental energy. Psychiatry Res 2006;148:195–203.

11 Bah J, Lindstrom M, Westberg L, et al: Serotonin transporter gene polymorphisms: effect on serotonin transporter availability in the brain of suicide attempters. Psychiatry Res 2008;162:221–229.

12 Oquendo MA, Hastings RS, Huang YY, et al: Brain serotonin transporter binding in depressed patients with bipolar disorder using positron emission tomography. Arch Gen Psychiatry 2007;64:201–208.

13 Parsey RV, Hastings RS, Oquendo MA, et al: Lower serotonin transporter binding potential in the human brain during major depressive episodes. Am J Psychiatry 2006;163:52–58.

14 van Heeringen C, Audenaert K, Van Laere K, et al: Prefrontal 5-HT_{2A} receptor binding index, hopelessness and personality characteristics in attempted suicide. J Affect Disord 2003;74:149–158.

15 Meyer JH, McMain S, Kennedy SH, et al: Dysfunctional attitudes and 5-HT2 receptors during depression and self-harm. Am J Psychiatry 2003;160:90–99.

16 Soloff PH, Price JC, Meltzer CC, Fabio A, Frank GK, Kaye WH: 5-HT_{2A} receptor binding is increased in borderline personality disorder. Biol Psychiatry 2007;62:580–587.

17 Leyton M, Paquette V, Gravel P, et al: α-[^{11}C]methyl-L-tryptophan trapping in the orbital and ventral medial prefrontal cortex of suicide attempters. Eur Neuropsychopharmacol 2006;16:220–223.

18 Li J, Kuang WH, Zou K, et al: A proton magnetic spectroscopy research on hippocampus metabolisms in people with suicide-attempted depressions (in Chinese). Sichuan Da Xue Xue Bao Yi Xue Ban 2009;40:59–62.

19 Zhong S, Wang Y, Zhao G, et al: Similarities of biochemical abnormalities between major depressive disorder and bipolar depression: a proton magnetic resonance spectroscopy study. J Affect Disord 2014;168:380–386.

20 Sachs-Ericsson N, Hames JL, Joiner TE, et al: Differences between suicide attempters and nonattempters in depressed older patients: depression severity, white-matter lesions, and cognitive functioning. Am J Geriatr Psychiatry 2014;22:75–85.

21 Ehrlich S, Noam GG, Lyoo IK, Kwon BJ, Clark MA, Renshaw PF: White matter hyperintensities and their associations with suicidality in psychiatrically hospitalized children and adolescents. J Am Acad Child Adolesc Psychiatry 2004;43:770–776.
22 Ehrlich S, Breeze JL, Hesdorffer DC, et al: White matter hyperintensities and their association with suicidality in depressed young adults. J Affect Disord 2005;86:281–287.
23 Pompili M, Ehrlich S, De Pisa E, et al: White matter hyperintensities and their associations with suicidality in patients with major affective disorders. Eur Arch Psychiatry Clin Neurosci 2007;257:494–499.
24 Pompili M, Innamorati M, Mann JJ, et al: Periventricular white matter hyperintensities as predictors of suicide attempts in bipolar disorders and unipolar depression. Prog Neuropsychopharmacol Biol Psychiatry 2008;32:1501–1507.
25 Mann JJ, Huang YY, Underwood MD, et al: A serotonin transporter gene promoter polymorphism (5-HTTLPR) and prefrontal cortical binding in major depression and suicide. Arch Gen Psychiatry 2000;57:729–738.
26 Benedetti F, Radaelli D, Poletti S, et al: Opposite effects of suicidality and lithium on gray matter volumes in bipolar depression. J Affect Disord 2011; 135:139–147.
27 Aguilar EJ, Garcia-Marti G, Marti-Bonmati L, et al: Left orbitofrontal and superior temporal gyrus structural changes associated to suicidal behavior in patients with schizophrenia. Prog Neuropsychopharmacol Biol Psychiatry 2008;32:1673–1676.
28 Monkul ES, Hatch JP, Nicoletti MA, et al: Fronto-limbic brain structures in suicidal and non-suicidal female patients with major depressive disorder. Mol Psychiatry 2007;12:360–366.
29 Giakoumatos CI, Tandon N, Shah J, et al: Are structural brain abnormalities associated with suicidal behavior in patients with psychotic disorders? J Psychiatr Res 2013;47:1389–1395.
30 Wagner G, Koch K, Schachtzabel C, Schultz CC, Sauer H, Schlosser RG: Structural brain alterations in patients with major depressive disorder and high risk for suicide: evidence for a distinct neurobiological entity? Neuroimage 2011;54:1607–1614.
31 Hwang JP, Lee TW, Tsai SJ, et al: Cortical and subcortical abnormalities in late-onset depression with history of suicide attempts investigated with MRI and voxel-based morphometry. J Geriatr Psychiatry Neurol 2010;23:171–184.
32 Goodman M, Hazlett EA, Avedon JB, Siever DR, Chu KW, New AS: Anterior cingulate volume reduction in adolescents with borderline personality disorder and co-morbid major depression. J Psychiatr Res 2011;45:803–807.
33 Rusch N, Spoletini I, Wilke M, et al: Inferior frontal white matter volume and suicidality in schizophrenia. Psychiatry Res 2008;164:206–214.
34 Soloff PH, Pruitt P, Sharma M, Radwan J, White R, Diwadkar VA: Structural brain abnormalities and suicidal behavior in borderline personality disorder. J Psychiatr Res 2012.
35 Wagner G, Schultz CC, Koch K, Schachtzabel C, Sauer H, Schlosser RG: Prefrontal cortical thickness in depressed patients with high risk for suicidal behavior. J Psychiatr Res 2012;46:1449–1455.
36 Baldacara L, Nery-Fernandes F, Rocha M, et al: Is cerebellar volume related to bipolar disorder? J Affect Disord 2011;135:305–309.
37 Dombrovski AY, Siegle GJ, Szanto K, Clark L, Reynolds CF, Aizenstein H: The temptation of suicide: striatal gray matter, discounting of delayed rewards, and suicide attempts in late-life depression. Psychol Med 2012;42:1203–1215.
38 Vang FJ, Ryding E, Traskman-Bendz L, van Westen D, Lindstrom MB: Size of basal ganglia in suicide attempters, and its association with temperament and serotonin transporter density. Psychiatry Res 2010; 183:177–179.
39 Lopez-Larson M, King JB, McGlade E, et al: Enlarged thalamic volumes and increased fractional anisotropy in the thalamic radiations in veterans with suicide behaviors. Front Psychiatry 2013;4:83.
40 Spoletini I, Piras F, Fagioli S, et al: Suicidal attempts and increased right amygdala volume in schizophrenia. Schizophr Res 2011;125:30–40.
41 Vythilingam M, Heim C, Newport J, et al: Childhood trauma associated with smaller hippocampal volume in women with major depression. Am J Psychiatry 2002;159:2072–2080.
42 Turecki G, Ernst C, Jollant F, Labonte B, Mechawar N: The neurodevelopmental origins of suicidal behavior. Trends Neurosci 2012;35:14–23.
43 Cyprien F, Courtet P, Malafosse A, et al: Suicidal behavior is associated with reduced corpus callosum area. Biol Psychiatry 2011;70:320–326.
44 Nery-Fernandes F, Rocha MV, Jackowski A, et al: Reduced posterior corpus callosum area in suicidal and non-suicidal patients with bipolar disorder. J Affect Disord 2012;142:150–155.
45 Matsuo K, Nielsen N, Nicoletti MA, et al: Anterior genu corpus callosum and impulsivity in suicidal patients with bipolar disorder. Neurosci Lett 2010;469: 75–80.
46 Jovev M, Garner B, Phillips L, et al: An MRI study of pituitary volume and parasuicidal behavior in teenagers with first-presentation borderline personality disorder. Psychiatry Res 2008;162:273–277.
47 Cipriani A, Hawton K, Stockton S, Geddes JR: Lithium in the prevention of suicide in mood disorders: updated systematic review and meta-analysis. BMJ 2013;346:f3646.

48 Jia Z, Huang X, Wu Q, et al: High-field magnetic resonance imaging of suicidality in patients with major depressive disorder. Am J Psychiatry 2010;67:1381–1390.

49 Jia Z, Wang Y, Huang X, et al: Impaired frontothalamic circuitry in suicidal patients with depression revealed by diffusion tensor imaging at 3.0 T. J Psychiatry Neurosci 2014;39:170–177.

50 Mahon K, Burdick KE, Wu J, Ardekani BA, Szeszko PR: Relationship between suicidality and impulsivity in bipolar I disorder: a diffusion tensor imaging study. Bipolar Disord 2012;14:80–89.

51 Olvet DM, Peruzzo D, Thapa-Chhetry B, et al: A diffusion tensor imaging study of suicide attempters. J Psychiatr Res 2014;51:60–67.

52 Richard-Devantoy S, Berlim MT, Jollant F: A meta-analysis of neuropsychological markers of vulnerability to suicidal behavior in mood disorders. Psychol Med 2014;44:1663–1674.

53 Jollant F, Lawrence NS, Olie E, et al: Decreased activation of lateral orbitofrontal cortex during risky choices under uncertainty is associated with disadvantageous decision-making and suicidal behavior. Neuroimage 2010;51:1275–1281.

54 Pan L, Segreti A, Almeida J, et al: Preserved hippocampal function during learning in the context of risk in adolescent suicide attempt. Psychiatry Res 2013;211:112–118.

55 Dombrovski AY, Szanto K, Clark L, Reynolds CF, Siegle GJ: Reward signals, attempted suicide, and impulsivity in late-life depression. JAMA Psychiatry 2013, Epub ahead of print.

56 Willeumier K, Taylor DV, Amen DG: Decreased cerebral blood flow in the limbic and prefrontal cortex using SPECT imaging in a cohort of completed suicides. Transl Psychiatry 2011;1:e28.

57 Amen DG, Prunella JR, Fallon JH, Amen B, Hanks C: A comparative analysis of completed suicide using high resolution brain SPECT imaging. J Neuropsychiatry Clin Neurosci 2009;21:430–439.

58 Pan LA, Batezati-Alves SC, Almeida JR, et al: Dissociable patterns of neural activity during response inhibition in depressed adolescents with and without suicidal behavior. J Am Acad Child Adolesc Psychiatry 2011;50:602–611.e3.

59 Audenaert K, Goethals I, Van Laere K, et al: SPECT neuropsychological activation procedure with the Verbal Fluency Test in attempted suicide patients. Nucl Med Commun 2002;23:907–916.

60 Jollant F, Lawrence NS, Giampietro V, et al: Orbitofrontal cortex response to angry faces in men with histories of suicide attempts. Am J Psychiatry 2008;165:740–748.

61 Pan LA, Hassel S, Segreti AM, Nau SA, Brent DA, Phillips ML: Differential patterns of activity and functional connectivity in emotion processing neural circuitry to angry and happy faces in adolescents with and without suicide attempt. Psychol Med 2013;43:2129–2142.

62 Schneidman ES: The Suicidal Mind. New York, Oxford University Press, 1996.

63 Reisch T, Seifritz E, Esposito F, Wiest R, Valach L, Michel K: An fMRI study on mental pain and suicidal behavior. J Affect Disord 2010;126:321–335.

64 Buckner RL, Andrews-Hanna JR, Schacter DL: The brain's default network: anatomy, function, and relevance to disease. Ann NY Acad Sci 2008;1124:1–38.

65 Fountoulakis KN, Iacovides A, Fotiou F, et al: Neurobiological and psychological correlates of suicidal attempts and thoughts of death in patients with major depression. Neuropsychobiology 2004;49:42–52.

66 Fan T, Wu X, Yao L, Dong J: Abnormal baseline brain activity in suicidal and non-suicidal patients with major depressive disorder. Neurosci Lett 2013;534:35–40.

67 Sublette ME, Milak MS, Galfalvy HC, Oquendo MA, Malone KM, Mann JJ: Regional brain glucose uptake distinguishes suicide attempters from non-attempters in major depression. Arch Suicide Res 2013;17:434–447.

68 van Heeringen K, Bijttebier S, Desmyter S, Vervaet M, Baeken C: Is there a neuroanatomical basis of the vulnerability to suicidal behavior? A coordinate-based meta-analysis of structural and functional MRI studies. Front Hum Neurosci 2014;8:824.

69 Richard-Devantoy S, Orsat M, Dumais A, Turecki G, Jollant F: Neurocognitive vulnerability: suicidal and homicidal behaviours in patients with schizophrenia. Can J Psychiatry 2014;59:18–25.

70 Jollant F, Lawrence NL, Olie E, Guillaume S, Courtet P: The suicidal mind and brain: a review of neuropsychological and neuroimaging studies. World J Biol Psychiatry 2011;12:319–339.

71 Szanto K, Clark L, Hallquist M, Vanyukov P, Crockett M, Dombrovski AY: The cost of social punishment and high-lethality suicide attempts in the second half of life. Psychol Aging 2014;29:84–94.

72 Jollant F, Guillaume S, Jaussent I, Castelnau D, Malafosse A, Courtet P: Impaired decision-making in suicide attempters may increase the risk of problems in affective relationships. J Affect Disord 2007;99:59–62.

73 Glascher J, Adolphs R, Damasio H, et al: Lesion mapping of cognitive control and value-based decision making in the prefrontal cortex. Proc Natl Acad Sci U S A 2012;109:14681–14686.

74 Richard-Devantoy S, Berlim MT, Jollant F: Suicidal behaviour and memory: a systematic review and meta-analysis. World J Biol Psychiatry 2014;1–23.

75 Ray RD, Ochsner KN, Cooper JC, Robertson ER, Gabrieli JD, Gross JJ: Individual differences in trait rumination and the neural systems supporting cognitive reappraisal. Cogn Affect Behav Neurosci 2005;5:156–168.

76 van Heeringen K, Van den Abbeele D, Vervaet M, Soenen L, Audenaert K: The functional neuroanatomy of mental pain in depression. Psychiatry Res 2010;181:141–144.

77 Moussa MN, Steen MR, Laurienti PJ, Hayasaka S: Consistency of network modules in resting-state fMRI connectome data. PLoS One 2012;7:e44428.

78 Arie M, Apter A, Orbach I, Yefet Y, Zalzman G: Autobiographical memory, interpersonal problem solving, and suicidal behavior in adolescent inpatients. Compr Psychiatry 2008;49:22–29.

Fabrice Jollant
Douglas Mental Health University Institute
6875 Boulevard LaSalle
Montreal, QC H4H 1R3 (Canada)
E-Mail fabrice.jollant@mcgill.ca

Kaschka WP, Rujescu D (eds): Biological Aspects of Suicidal Behavior.
Adv Biol Psychiatry. Basel, Karger, 2016, vol 30, pp 123–144 (DOI: 10.1159/000434746)

Inflammation and Suicidal Behavior

Teodor T. Postolache[a–c] · Partam Manalai[d] · Lisa A. Brenner[e–g] · Lena Brundin[h, i]

[a]Department of Psychiatry, University of Maryland-Baltimore School of Medicine, and [b]Veterans Integrated Service Network (VISN) 5, Mental Illness Research Education and Clinical Center (MIRECC), Baltimore, Md., [c]Rocky Mountain, Mental Illness Research Education and Clinical Center (MIRECC), Denver, Colo., [d]Department of Psychiatry, Howard University, Washington, D.C., Departments of [e]Psychiatry, [f]Physical Medicine and Rehabilitation and [g]Neurology, University of Colorado, Anschutz Medical Campus, Aurora, Colo., [h]Division of Psychiatry and Behavioral Medicine, College of Human Medicine, Michigan State University, and [i]Van Andel Research Institute, Grand Rapids, Mich., USA

Abstract

Clinical and epidemiological data accumulated over the past decade strongly suggest that inflammation, certain upstream triggers of the immune system and downstream molecular mediators of inflammation, may contribute to the pathophysiology of suicidal behavior. Upstream factors include autoimmune factors, infections, traumatic brain injury, and stress. Downstream factors potentially mediating the effects of inflammation include molecules of the kynurenine pathway, which are known to modulate neuroinflammation and glutamate neurotransmission. The following could contribute to an important rejuvenation of our suicide prevention arsenal: (1) targeting immune dysregulation in patients with a history of suicidal behavior; (2) preventive factors involving upstream activators such as chronic latent infections or allergens and, (3) interrupting downstream pathophysiological pathways of inflammation. Additionally, the focus on individual triggers and diatheses will increase the precision of our treatment interventions in suicide prevention. Finally, it might be possible to increase the accuracy of suicide risk estimation by adding analysis of inflammatory biomarkers to our clinical information and neuropsychological testing. Discovering novel agents that target inflammation may also rejuvenate our therapeutic interval in suicide prevention.

Death by suicide is the 14th cause of years of life lost [1], with at least 1 million deaths every year [2]. If current trends continue, it is expected that annually at least 1.5 million lives will be ended prematurely by suicide in 2020 [3]. The burden of suicidal behavior includes the economic and emotional impact of suicide on survivors and the high frequency of attempts (10–20 times more frequent than suicides). Despite recent progress in utilizing certain treatment options for suicidal behavior, including lithium in mood disorders, clozapine in schizophrenia and possibly electroconvulsive treatment in treatment-resistant depression, suicide rates have been increasing in the USA. As such, it is imperative to continue improving detection, prevention and management of suicidal behavior.

One area with the most replicated biological findings implicated in suicidal behavior involve changes in the hypothalamic-pituitary-adrenal (HPA) axis activity [4], as well as serotonergic transmission [4, 5]. Both HPA axis activities and serotoninergic neurotransmission have reciprocal interactions with the immune system, centrally and peripherally.

Risk Factors for Suicide

Complex interactions [6] between genetic predispositions and environmental factors are thought to drive suicidal behavior (including death by suicide and suicide attempts). The best predictor of a future suicide is a history of attempts [7]. Psychiatric disorders, in particular major depression and bipolar disorder, frequently co-occur among those who die by suicide [8].

Sickness Behavior

Activation of the immune system profoundly impacts mammals. A 'sickness' behavioral syndrome describes behavioral changes induced by infection or other inflammatory triggers [9]. Peripherally produced immune mediators, such as cytokines, can reach the CNS via blood (crossing an inflamed and thus more permeable blood-brain barrier, BBB, or through areas where the BBB is lacking – such as structures called circumventricular organs). Alternatively, cytokines can bypass the BBB by using the pathway of cranial nerves (e.g. vagus, olfactory, trigeminal nerves) or through the lumen or walls of vascular structures. The translocation of immune mediators from periphery to CNS, or the constitutional production of mediators in the CNS, often augmented by peripheral immune stimuli, do not always have negative consequences. In fact the constitutional production of cytokines secreted by microglia, endothelial cells and astrocytes plays an important role in CNS maintenance and development [10]. During episodes of inflammation triggered sickness, cytokine-induced sickness behavior, which is responsible for channeling resources to survival and overcoming infection, and thus changes in sleep and sleepiness, reduction in appetite, food intake, reduced interest in exploring the environment and sex are evolutionarily intertwined with survival.

Clinically, while there are similarities between sickness and depression, especially in regard to neurovegetative symptoms, there are marked differences concerning the individual's regard for the present, the future, the past, and self. Specifically, helplessness, hopelessness, guilt, worthlessness, and suicidal ideation (active or passive) do not belong to the syndrome of sickness and point towards depression, requiring treatment.

Inflammation, Depression and Other Psychiatric Conditions

Increasing evidence links inflammation to symptoms of depression. For instance, dysphoria and anxiety can be triggered by the induction of inflammation, with microbial triggers below the threshold concentrations allowing the induction of sickness behavior and a secondary psychological reaction to it [11]. Medical conditions with known immune mediation such as systemic lupus erythematous, multiple sclerosis and traumatic brain injury (TBI) are associated with markedly increased prevalence rates of depression. Individuals with autoimmune conditions and certain infections have increased blood markers of inflammation and are also at risk for developing different types of mood disorders, including bipolar disorder [12]. Markers [13] of inflammation, including C-reactive protein (CRP), IL-6 and TNF-α, have often been found to be increased in patients with MDD [14]. Similarly, treatment for hepatitis C with IFN-α induces depression in a subgroup of patients [15]. It has been reported that levels of proinflammatory cytokines correlate with depressive symptoms [16, 17]. Similarly, several meta-analyses have confirmed abnormal levels of immune markers, including cytokines [18, 19] and CRP [20], in patients with bipolar disorders. Slightly elevated CRP levels of between 3 and 10 mg/l are useful for the concept of 'low-grade inflammation' that has been associated with conditions that increase the risk of suicide such as schizophrenia [21], anxiety disorders [22], depression [21], and bipolar disorder [20].

Is the association between inflammation and mood disorder a trait or state finding? Results are mixed and tend to suggest that certain associations tend to represent trait markers, others state markers and others 'scars', i.e. consequences of being exposed to prior episodes. In a recent meta-analysis, the CRP values tended to 'normalize' during the depressed phase of bipolar disorder and to appear elevated during the manic and euthymic phases of patients [20].

Neuroimaging techniques have evolved enabling us to improve our ability to distinguish state inflammation. For instance, positron emission tomography (PET) can be used to quantify translocator protein (TSPO) binding, a mitochondrial protein of microglial origin, which increases during neuroinflammation, when microglia become activated [23]. Novel tracers have been developed to bind to TSPO [24, 25]. Two recent studies have underscored the importance of state rather than trait in studying low-grade inflammation in the brain. A negative study [26] investigated TSPO binding in patients in heterogeneous states (treated vs. untreated, symptomatic vs. minimally symptomatic). In contrast, when all patients were investigated during a symptomatic major depressive episode, with all patients medication free for at least six weeks, significant elevations of TSPO distribution volume were identified in the prefrontal cortex, anterior cingulate cortex and insula [27]. More specifically, a greater severity of depression correlated with TSPO distribution volume in the anterior cingulate cortex – a brain region previously implicated in the modulation of emotional and behavioral expression of depression.

Inflammation and Suicidal Ideation and Behavior

The development of suicidal ideation and attempts has been also reported in immunotherapy trials [28, 29]. In particular, during and after treatment with IFN-β, suicide ideation and attempts have emerged in previously psychiatrically healthy individuals [30]. To our knowledge, a report by Nassberger and Traskman-Bendz [31] (1993) on increased values of soluble IL-2 receptor was the first to document cytokine elevations in patients with a history of suicide attempt. After more than 15 years, a study by Postolache (author in this article) and colleagues [32] at the University of Maryland (2008) found increased mRNA transcription of anti-inflammatory cytokines IL-4 and IL-13 in the orbitofrontal cortex of suicide victims. This was particularly relevant, as this elevation was reported in an area involved in affective and behavioral modulation and an area where histopathological changes involving serotonin terminals had previously been reported [4]. The elevation of anti-inflammatory cytokine gene expression could be seen as compensatory, in the effort of tuning down inflammation triggered by associated mental states that led to the fatal attempt, including depression, anguish and stress. The same year Steiner et al. [33] found significant microgliosis in suicide cases diagnosed with schizophrenia and depression compared with individuals with the same diagnoses who died from causes other than suicide. A number of studies led by coauthor Brundin and colleagues [34] that took place at Lund University identified elevations of IL-6 in the cerebrospinal fluid (CSF) of suicide attempters. They reported elevations in plasma IL-6 and TNF-α in the plasma from suicide attempters compared with both healthy controls and depressed nonsuicidal patients [35]. In contrast, a decreased production of IL-6 (and IL-2) by whole blood immune stimulation in a culture setting was documented in patients with suicidal depression compared with patients with nonsuicidal MDD [36].

A similarly unexpected finding was reported by Gabbay et al. [37], who found lower plasma TNF-α levels in adolescents with suicidal depression compared with nonsuicidal adolescents with MDD. Either peripheral levels of TNF-α may not accurately reflect brain levels of the cytokines or immune responses in completed suicide may differ from those with nonfatal suicidal behavior, as, in the postmortem prefrontal cortex of adolescent suicides, Pandey et al. [38] (2012) reported increased levels of mRNA and protein levels for TNF-α, as well as other proinflammatory cytokines IL-1β and IL-6. Moreover, protein S-100B, a marker of CNS inflammation, was reported to be positively associated with the severity of suicidal ideation in adolescents diagnosed with depression or psychotic disorder [39]. A more recent study identified an association of suicidal ideation with 'inflammatory index', including levels of CRP and cytokines IL-6, TNF-α and IL-10, independent of recent history of attempt and severity of depression [40], making a potential contribution to developing 'latent variables' in mediation analyses using structural equation modeling.

An important recent meta-analysis on blood, CSF and postmortem tissue findings concluded that cytokines could successfully distinguish individuals with lethal and nonlethal suicidal behavior from nonsuicidal patients. Increased levels of IL-1β and IL-6 in blood and postmortem samples, decreased production of IL-2 by peripheral mononuclear cells and decreased CSF IL-8 levels stood out as the most relevant immune biomarkers distinguishing suicidal behavior from nonsuicidal behaviors [41]. In a systematic review on inflammation in relation to suicidal behavior, Serafini et al. [42] concluded that immune markers can distinguish patients with depression versus without suicidal ideation/attempts but that this association remains a simple associative rather than predictive link in the absence of longitudinal studies. A recent study on blood biomarkers concluded that markers of the biological pathways of inflammation, apoptosis and stress may represent important convergent pathophysiological pathways of suicidal ideation and suicide [43].

Downstream Factors

Constitutive Expression of Cytokines and Direct Effects

Cytokine receptors are presented in areas involved in mood regulation and dysregulation, including areas of the prefrontal cortex, hippocampus and cerebellum and in the raphe neurons in the medulla oblongata [44, 45]. The neurons of the amygdala, thalamus and hippocampus and 5-HT_2 receptor-expressing neurons in the hypothalamus have IL-1β receptors [46]. These receptors underlie important physiological functions of constitutive cytokines in brain physiology. For instance, IL-6, IL-1β and TNF-α have been implicated in the regulation of synaptic plasticity and transmission [47, 48] in normal conditions and after immune challenge [49, 50]. Cytokines have been shown to alter levels of metabolites of monoaminergic neurotransmitters as well as their levels in different regions of the CNS involved in behavioral modulation or moderation.

See figure 1 for downstream factors translating the effect of inflammation on brain structure and function.

Associations with Intermediate Phenotypes of Suicidal Behavior

Aggression, helplessness [51] and impulsivity have been proposed as intermediate phenotypes of suicidal behavior [52]. In humans, there have been studies confirming associations between aggression and anger with inflammation. For instance, anger is positively associated with IL-6 levels [53] and, in patients with self-harm, hostility is

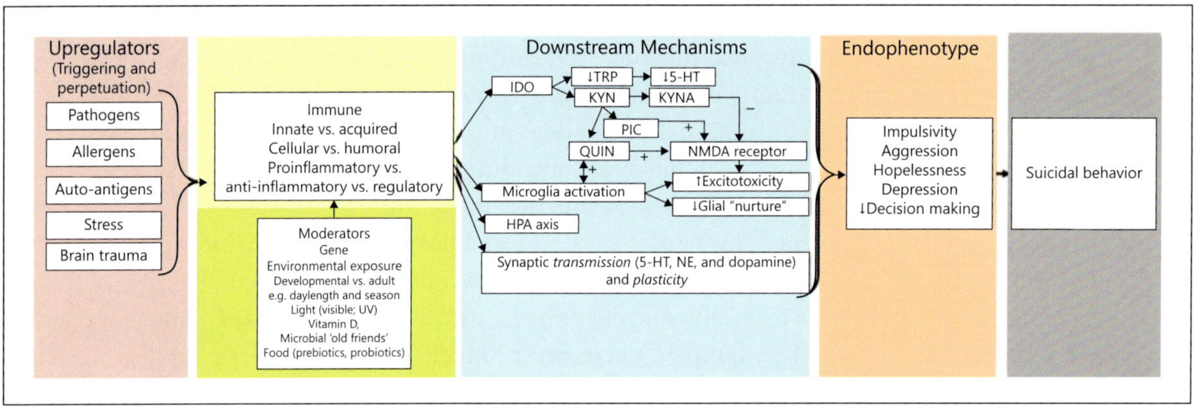

Fig. 1. Immune factors, their upstream upregulation, their downstream mechanisms related to suicidal behavior, risk factors, and intermediate phenotypes, and their moderators. 5-HT = Serotonin; NE = norepinephrine; KYN = kynurenine; PIC = picolinic acid.

associated with elevations in IL-1β [54]. Hostility and anger were also found to be increased during IFN-α treatment of hepatitis C [55], with moderation of this effect by a specific genetic variability in the TNF-α gene [56]. However, it is the animal research that has advanced this knowledge towards causation. For instance, aggressive behaviors in cats have been precipitated by an injection of IL-1β into the medial hypothalamus or periaqueductal gray, via 5-HT_2 receptors [57, 58]. The effects of IL-2 injected into the periaqueductal gray appear to be mediated by NK_1 receptors [59]. Moreover, it appears that aggression regulation requires TNF-α, as TNF-α receptor-deficient mice do not react aggressively in a resident intruder test, a common animal paradigm to quantify aggressive-like behavior [60].

The Kynurenine Pathway

Another downstream mechanism that could impact the behavioral and emotional regulation implicated in suicidal behavior is the activation of tryptophan breakdown via the kynurenine pathway (fig. 1). In fact, enzymatic aberrations on this path have been proposed to be a main mechanism leading away from inflammation-induced 'uncomplicated' sickness behavior towards depression and suicidality [9, 61]. Proinflammatory cytokines, predominantly IFN-γ but also, to a lesser degree, IL-6 and IL-1β induce the enzymes indoleamine 2,3-dioxygenase (IDO-1) and, secondarily, tryptophan 2,3-dioxygenase (TDO-2), the first steps of initiating the kynurenine pathway [62, 63]. Through shifting tryptophan breakdown through the kynurenine pathway, the resulting tryptophan depletion may further induce a decrease in levels of serotonin and potentially decreased levels of serotonin metabolite found in those with a history of nonfatal suicidal self-directed violence [64]. The serotonin depletion secondary to the activation of IDO by inflammation remains a theoretical construct, as it has not been yet proven by empirical evidence.

Activation of the kynurenine pathway produces several neuroactive compounds, including the excitotoxic quinolinic acid (QUIN) and neuroprotective kynurenic acid (KYNA) [65]. Importantly, over 90% of tryptophan degradation occurs in the periphery [66], with enzymes of this pathway found in a multitude of cells, including immune cells, brain, liver, and kidney. In the brain, a cellular segregation of the kynurenine metabolism QUIN, N-methyl-D-aspartic acid (NMDA) receptors containing the NR1 + NR2A and the NR1 + NR2B subunits [67, 68], occurs predominantly in microglial cells. QUIN has convergent excitotoxic potency, elevating glutamatergic neurotransmission through several mechanisms. Beyond its NMDA agonism, QUIN also increases neuronal glutamate release and decreases glutamate uptake and recycling by astrocytes [69]. KYNA, produced predominantly in astrocytes, is an antagonist at the glycine site of the NMDA receptor and a blocker of the cholinergic α-7 nicotinic receptor (α-7nAChR). KYNA has neuroprotective properties and anticonvulsive effects but may contribute to cognitive deficits and, in particular, its elevation is predictively associated with schizophrenia [70, 71].

The collaboration of coauthor Postolache with John Mann's group [72] at Columbia University led to the first study reporting abnormalities of the kynurenine pathway in relation to suicidal behavior, specifically elevated plasma kynurenine levels in patients with depression who attempted suicide compared with depressed patients with no history of self-directed violence. Kynurenine passes freely through the BBB and into the brain and, although inactive, initiates the production of neuroactive metabolites [65].

In collaboration, coauthors Brundin and Postolache and group [73] have reported elevations of QUIN in suicide attempters to more than twice those in healthy controls, while levels of KYNA were not different from controls, and thus produced a higher QUIN/KYNA quotient in suicide attempters. The likelihood of the production of QUIN by ongoing low-grade inflammation has been supported by positive correlations between CSF QUIN and CSF IL-6 levels. QUIN elevations in suicide attempters were positively associated with high suicide intent scores and were predominantly 'state dependent'. A follow-up study reported CSF QUIN levels as elevated in suicide attempters in comparison with healthy controls also as a trait, albeit to a lower degree than in the immediate temporal proximity of a suicide attempt [74]. Higher cytokine levels and lower CSF KYNA levels were positively associated with the magnitude of depressive symptoms and suicidality scores. In line with this finding, a previous study reported lower blood KYNA levels in patients with depression [75], consistent also with a lower neuroprotective/neurotoxic KYNA/QUIN ratio in bipolar patients relative to healthy controls [76]. While a more recent brain imaging study did not replicate the lower value of KYNA in patients with major depression, it was nevertheless positively associated with hippocampal and amygdala volume in those patients, probably through the neuroprotective effects of KYNA [77]. Indeed, a reduction in dendritic growth secondary to neuronal exposure to extracellular glutamate is prevented by the administration of

KYNA [78]. Additionally, experimental work suggests that an inhibitor of kynurenine-3-monooxygenase, minimizing the production of QUIN and elevating the production of KYNA, reverses the inhibitory effects of IL-1 on hippocampal neurogenesis [79].

Van Heeringen et al. [80] (2014) proposed that increased levels of QUIN, through neurotoxicity, could contribute to structural loss and cell loss in brain regions previously described in individuals with suicidal behavior. This is consistent with postmortem data reporting increase counts of QUIN-reactive microglia in the anterior midcingulate cortex and the subgenual anterior cingulate cortex [81]. Taking into account the convergent clinical, imaging and postmortem literature towards a neurotoxic QUIN balanced by neuroprotective KYNA in suicidal behavior, the very high levels of glutamate agonist QUIN in suicide attempters in temporal proximity of attempt [73] provide a rationale for clinical trials of ketamine, an NMDA receptor antagonist showing rapid resolution of suicidal ideation [82, 83] in individuals at risk with elevated QUIN/KYNA ratios.

Upstream Factors Associated with Inflammation and Suicidal Behavior

Toxoplasma gondii

T. gondii, a widespread neurotropic protozoan parasite, infects approximately a third of all humans. Symptoms of infection range from none to minimal depending on the adequacy of the host immune response [84]. Congenital infection, occurring if a mother has a primary infection during pregnancy and passes it to the fetus, though calamitous, is relatively rare. Within the animal world, felids have been identified as the definitive host to *T. gondii*. *T. gondii* may infect humans via ingestion of the parasite's oocysts, which can spread from the feces of infected cats. Other routes of transmission include consumption of undercooked meat that has been infected with *T. gondii* cysts or ingestion of contaminated water. When ingested by an intermediate host, the parasite spreads from the intestine to other organs, finally localizing in muscle and brain. In the brain, *T. gondii* hides within neurons and glial cells, forming intracellular characteristic cystic structures. Latent toxoplasmosis, the asymptomatic persistence of cysts in host tissues, including the brain, is prevalent in 25–30% of the global population [85], with a relatively lower prevalence (10–15%) reported in the USA [86]. Prevalence is higher among those who lived or live in rural areas. Approximately 60 million men, women and children in the USA carry *T. gondii* [86]. Latent toxoplasmosis has been associated with subclinical personality traits [87–89], subtle neurological deficits [90] and a heightened risk of motor vehicle accidents [91], as well as major psychiatric illness such as schizophrenia [92], bipolar disorder [93] and personality disorders [94]. Intermittent reactivation of latent infection of *T. gondii* has been previously proposed to explain psychiatric manifestations in immunosuppressed patients [95, 96].

T. gondii Increases 'Risk Taking'

In rodents, latent *T. gondii* infection reduces and even reverses innate fear of cat odor and other stimuli that precede predation [97]. Although some mixed findings have been noted, *T. gondii* infection has also been found to nonspecifically lower fear/anxiety and increase novelty seeking in rodents [98–100]. Certain immunological parameters associated with suicidal behavior are among the very ones involved in the protection against brain invasion by *T. gondii* such as cytokines TNF-α, IL-6 and microglia activation. Conversely, mechanisms of immune manipulation by the parasite can induce the production of anti-inflammatory cytokines that reduce the ability to clear the microorganism [101].

T. gondii and Suicidal Behavior

Our work in support of this relationship includes cross-sectional studies of mood disorders [102], a study of German patients with schizophrenia [103], an ecological study in Europe [104], and a prospective cohort study in Danish mothers [105]. Results from a Swedish cohort highlighted convergent evidence for the hypothesized association between *T. gondii* and suicide attempts [106]. These findings were replicated by independent groups in Turkey among those with a history of attempt [107] and young adults in Poland [108]. Specifically, seropositivity rates were 71% in the suicide group versus 44.4% in the control group ($p < 0.05$ in younger victims). This strong effect in younger patients is consistent with our study among schizophrenia patients [103]. In our study among those with mood disorders, serointensity rather than seropositivity was associated with a history of attempts [102]. This was replicated by a very recent study [109] (serointensity rather than seropositivity). Overall, the effect sizes have been higher when attempts were well documented [105] or confirmed in terms of intent [106] among those who died by suicide [108] rather than self-reported attempts [102, 103]. Lethality or violent attempt status also appears to strengthen the association [105, 106].

T. gondii and Intermediate Phenotypes of Aggression and Impulsivity

Collaborative work by some of the coauthors established associations between chronic infection with *T. gondii* and aggression and impulsivity traits (gender and age specific) in healthy individuals and between *T. gondii* and aggression in patients with intermittent explosive disorder. A study of *T. gondii* association with trait aggression and impulsivity in healthy adults (collaboration of Postolache, Brenner and Brundin with Dr. Rujescu and colleagues [110] from Halle University) involved 1,000 community-residing adults residing in the Munich metropolitan area with no axis I or II conditions by SCID for DSM-IV (510 men, 490 women, mean age 53.6 ± 15.8 years, range 20–74). Plasma samples were tested for IgG antibodies to *T. gondii,* HSV-1 and CMV by ELISA. Self-reported ratings of trait aggression scores (Questionnaire for Measuring Factors of Aggression, FAF) and trait impulsivity (Sensation-Seeking Scale-V, SSS-V) were analyzed by *T. gondii* seropositivity status.

Parallel analyses were performed for both HSV-1 and CMV to determine whether the observed effects for *T. gondii* were agent specific. *T. gondii* IgG seropositivity was significantly associated with higher trait reactive aggression scores among women ($p < 0.01$) but not among men. *T. gondii* positivity was also associated with higher impulsive sensation seeking (SSS-V disinhibition) among younger men ($p < 0.01$) aged 20–59 years (median age = 60). All associations with HSV-1 and CMV were not significant. The generalizability of the study is limited by its focus on healthy individuals with no psychiatric history. However, its design reduces the possibility that the observed associations with aggression and impulsivity are simply a consequence of previously reported connections between *T. gondii* and underlying psychiatric illness. In conclusion, the two later preliminary studies suggest strong associations between trait impulsivity/aggression and *T. gondii* infection in otherwise healthy individuals, as well as in psychiatric patients with a tendency towards impulsive aggression. In a study of aggressive/impulsive individuals (a collaboration of author Postolache with professor Coccaro and colleagues [111] from the University of Chicago), 358 physically healthy subjects participated in the study, with 110 healthy controls having no evidence of any psychiatric diagnosis,138 psychiatric controls meeting criteria for a lifetime diagnosis of a psychiatric disorder, but not for a lifetime diagnosis of intermittent explosive disorder, and 110 subjects meeting criteria for a lifetime diagnosis of intermittent explosive disorder. Aggression was assessed with the aggression score from the Life History of Aggression Assessment and the aggression (physical and verbal) score from the Buss-Perry Aggression Questionnaire. Impulsivity was assessed using the Barratt Impulsivity Scale [112] and the impulsivity scale from the Eysenck Personality Inventory-2 (EPQ-2). The actual history of aggression was also quantified and used to integrate in an aggression score. Aggression scores were significantly higher in *T. gondii* seropositive participants ($F_{1, 342} = 5.32$, $p = 0.022$). Impulsivity scores were also higher in seropositive *T. gondii* individuals ($F_{1, 325} = 3.83$, $p = 0.051$). However, associations with aggression remained significant after adjustment for impulsivity, while adjustment for impulsivity rendered the associations with aggression statistically insignificant.

Interconnections between *T. gondii* and the KYN Pathways

The production of IFN-γ and the activation of IDO represent major inhibitory mechanisms of *T. gondii* [113], as demonstrated in vitro [113] and in vivo [114]. *T. gondii* infection induces persistent brain elevations in kynurenine and its metabolite QUIN [114]. We hypothesized that *T. gondii* association with suicide attempt history would be stronger in those with high kynurenine levels. In 950 patients with schizophrenia, anti-*T. gondii* IgG antibodies were assayed with ELISA. The hypothesis was confirmed, as only those with kynurenine levels in the upper 25th percentile were associated with suicide attempts ($p < 0.01$). A direct immunosuppressive effect of high kynurenine concentrations can occur through the induction of apoptosis and regulatory T cell (Treg) differentiation in lymphocyte populations [115]. Kynurenine causes a predominant downregulatory apoptosis of effector T cells, most notably Th1 cells [116–120]. Dendritic cell immunogenicity is also downregulated via a kynurenine-dependent mechanism [121]. This inhibitory effect of kynurenine is mediated by the aryl hydrocarbon receptor [122] centrally involved in the generation of Treg at the expense of Th17 cells [122]. Clinically, expression of IDO has been implicated in immune evasion in cancer [123, 124] with a particular direct role of kynurenine in suppressing antitumor immune responses via the aryl hydrocarbon receptor [125]. It is possible that, specifically, while *T. gondii* induces IFN-α and triggers the induction of the kynurenine pathway with the initial production of kynurenine, in certain individuals the constitutional tendency for a higher production of kynurenine will then suppress the immune response, leading to more frequent and persistent *T. gondii* reactivation. Therefore, we postulate that high kynurenine levels elevate the risk of suicide attempt in *T. gondii*-infected individuals through immune activation and secondary QUIN production and NMDA-driven excitotoxity/apoptosis, alternating, in those with a tendency to overproduce kynurenine, with intermittent kynurenine-induced immunosuppression and reactivation of the parasite, potentially by dopamine production by the microorganism, considering its enzymatic endowment [126].

Allergens and Seasonal Pathogens

Seasonal peaks of suicide are highly replicated epidemiologically across continents, hemispheres and regions [127–133]. The most reliable seasonal trigger is change in photoperiod, although many factors have been considered in this association, including sunshine, photoperiod, weather and climate, and seasonal variation in socioeconomical factors and availability of means. Postolache et al. [131] at the University of Maryland started a systematic investigation of seasonal factors that may be immune mediated.

Certain respiratory and digestive infections have seasonal peaks, many of them just prior to the peaks of suicide. Influenza is highly seasonal, with peaks at the end of winter and spring. Okusaga et al. [134] (2010) reported that seropositivity for influenza B was associated with a history of attempt in patients with recurrent mood disorders, while higher seropositivity for influenza A and B and coronaviruses distinguished patients with recurrent mood disorders and healthy controls.

Considering the massive 'tsunamis' in atmospheric pollen in spring, Postolache et al. [135] from the University of Maryland School of Medicine have hypothesized that inflammatory signals induced by pollen could affect brain structure and function. In the first study in the USA they uncovered an association between relative rates of suicide in women and tree pollen counts. While not replicating their findings in a subsequent time interval in the USA [136], they did replicate it in Denmark, this time in both genders in collaboration with Qin et al. [137] from Aarhus University. The group went further to dissect components of this association at postmortem, animal and clinical levels.

First they identified allergy-related cytokines expressed in regions of the brain previously implicated in suicide, with higher levels of mRNA for these cytokines in suicides than in those who died of other causes [32]. Second, the group found these allergy-related cytokines to have increased expression in rodents sensitized and exposed to allergens [138]. Third, the group identified that rodents exposed to allergens manifested elevation anxiety-like behavior [138] as well as aggression after stress [139], with both anxiety and aggression being considered as risk factors for suicidal behavior. Fourth, Postolache and colleagues [140] reported pharmacoepidemiologically that prescriptions of intranasal corticosteroids, known to reduce cytokine production in the nose, were associated with lower suicide rates, while second-generation antihistamines, which induce symptomatic improvement without lowering cytokine production, were associated with a slightly elevated suicide rates. Fifth, intersecting aeroallergen exposure and allergen-specific IgE identified an interaction between a diathesis (allergen-specific IgE and history of mood disorder) and trigger (a specific allergen [141]) – potentially explaining why only some patients with allergy manifest worsening in suicide risk factors and only some patients with mood disorders exacerbate during exposure to aeroallergens. Sixth, the group also dissected the potential of allergic rhinitis to be confounded by asthma, and asthma has its own distinct association with suicide [142]. The asthma associations with suicide are much more inclusive than through allergy, e.g. iatrogenic-systemic corticosteroids often used to treat its exacerbations may elevate the risk of the exacerbation of an underlying mood disorder. However, the exacerbations of asthma tend to occur late in fall and winter, when there is generally a trough of suicide, rather than in spring. Moreover, even when only patients with allergic rhinitis are considered, i.e. when asthma patients are omitted, the associations with suicide remain significant but of a smaller degree [143].

Ongoing studies (e.g. collaboration between Cook and Postolache with researchers from Hungary) confirmed allergen-suicide associations. Another seasonal factor contributing to suicide that is potentially mediated by immune factors is air pollution. For instance, Kim et al. [144] reported that the rate of suicide in Korea (a country with particularly high suicide rates) was associated with levels of ambient particulate matter two days prior to suicide. As particulate matter contains abundant lipopolysaccharide, it is relevant that lipopolysaccharide administered intranasally results in depressive-like behaviors, increased cytokine gene expression in the prefrontal cortex and activation of the HPA axis at least as pronounced as the intraperitoneal administration (if not more so) [145].

The airborne intranasal immune triggers – microbes, allergens, pollutants – and the reactions to them have a potential to reach the brain via preferential pathways potentially bypassing the BBB. These pathways are reviewed by Tonelli et al. [145] and Postolache et al. [146], who also mention that sleep impairment, a documented suicide risk factor, could also be a partial mediator of the link between allergic rhinitis and suicidal behavior [147].

Vitamin D and Suicide

Vitamin D can be considered a hormone released into circulation and it is transported to target organs via a vitamin D binding protein. Vitamin D is also a 'vitamin' as, at least in temperate regions, exposure to UVB radiation and food intake fail to provide adequate amounts from mid-autumn to mid-spring. In consequence, hypovitaminosis D is very common in industrialized countries such as the USA [148].

Vitamin D deficiency is widespread, in particular at the end of winter and beginning of spring [149]. While it was previously thought that vitamin D 1α-hydroxylase, the limiting enzyme involved in the formation of the active form of vitamin D, $1{,}25(OH)_2D$, is only present in the kidney and liver, it has been shown that the enzyme is found in the brain [150], along with many other tissues. Similarly, the vitamin D receptors are found to be widely distributed, including in the CNS [151].

The older knowledge that vitamin D has strong effects on immune cells [152] has recently been more magnified, as low levels of vitamin D have been shown to exacerbate immune-mediated symptoms in animal models of autoimmune disease such as rheumatoid arthritis, systemic lupus erythematous, type I diabetes mellitus and inflammatory bowel disease [153]. Hypovitaminosis D also reduces the effectiveness of infection-containing immune responses, resulting in increased risk for tuberculosis [154] and, potentially, influenza [155]. In addition to effects on innate immunity (dendritic cells and macrophages [156]), the CD4-positive T lymphocytes (Th1, Th2, Th17, and Trigs) have been a preferred target of activated vitamin D. Specifically, $1{,}25(OH)_2D$ inhibits the Th1 cells and the production of Th1 cytokines and upregulates the Th2 cells and levels of Th2 cytokines Th17 cells; the production of Il-17 and Il-6 is also inhibited [157]. Tregs are strongly stimulated by activated Vitamin D [158].

Together with the genetic endocrinologist E. Streeten and colleagues [159], author Postolache proposed that lower vitamin D levels at the beginning of spring may be contributory to an increased seasonal risk for suicide, a hypothesis confirmed in a recent case-control study in the US military [160]. Moreover, the authors proposed that, considering associations of very low vitamin D with several major suicide risk factors, low vitamin D independent of season may be predictively associated with suicide. This was confirmed in the US military study of Umhau et al. [160]. Importantly, the relationship between 25(OH)D level and mortality was not linear, as increased odds of suicide were elevated only in the deficient range (<15 ng/ml), the range where immune abnormalities appear to be most important in vitro, ex vivo and in vivo. Another study from author Brundin and group [161] in Lund reported an association between low 25(OH)D levels and history of suicide attempts, as well as elevations in proinflammatory cytokines. Thus, it is highly conceivable that low vitamin D may contribute to both low-grade inflammation and, through reduced efficiency of immune response, more frequent and severe reactivation of chronic infection. This is currently under investigation. Longitudinal and interventional studies are necessary to tease apart the directions of causality of this vitamin D-immune suicide link with considerable preventative potential.

Autoimmunity and Suicidal Behavior

An elevation in suicide risk factors has been reported in a number of autoimmune conditions. For instance, in systemic lupus erythematosus and multiple sclerosis the rates of depression reach about 40% [162, 163]. In systemic lupus erythematosus, activation of microglia, abnormalities include dysfunction of the BBB, with increased permeability to mediators of inflammation and direct antibodies against the NMDA receptor [164]. In multiple sclerosis, the prototype autoimmune neurological condition, the suicide rate is more than doubled compared with the general population, as shown in a large study on 12,000 hospitalized multiple sclerosis patients [165], which was confirmed by a smaller study in Denmark [166]. A similar doubling of suicide risk was also reported for patients with celiac disease in Sweden – the result of a large study on 29,000 patients with the inflammatory condition [167]. However, a recent research study by Okusaga et al. [168] in collaboration with Dan Rujescu from Halle University did not find any significant elevation in the history of suicide attempt in patients with schizophrenia with positive antigliadin IgG antibodies compared with seronegatives (unpubl. data).

Traumatic Brain Injury

Based on a large study in Sweden, comparing death records in 200,000 individuals with TBI with 2 million controls, individuals with TBI have a 3-fold higher probability of dying from suicide [169]. TBI is a major factor in triggering immune activation in the brain. After brain trauma, microglial cells respond almost immediately and secrete proinflammatory cytokines [170]. A slightly delayed astrocyte activation follows [171]. While the activation of microglia is most often protective and restorative, the exaggerated and/or prolonged elevation in proinflammatory cytokines may contribute to secondary tissue damage [172] or neuronal death [173] and neuronal hyperexcitability [174]. TBI patients have significantly higher TNF-α levels than healthy controls, with levels positively associated with both suicidal ideation 12 months after injury and behavioral disinhibition [175]. TBI is associated with elevated kynurenine pathway activation [176]. Thus, based on data previously presented, it is possible that inflammation after TBI mediates the link between TBI and suicidal behavior.

Stress and Inflammation

Evidence has accumulated that not only classical immune triggers but also acute stress upregulates the proinflammatory cytokine IL-1β [177, 178]. This has been confirmed in multiple stress paradigms, most convincingly after a Trier Social Stress Test (TSST), a commonly used laboratory stress test involving mental arithmetic, speech giving and social threat [179–181]. TNF-α, previously elevated in the plasma of patients with a history of suicide attempts [35], also rises after the TSST [180, 181] as well as following other acute stressors [182, 183]. IL-6, also elevated in patients with a history of suicidal self-directed violence, as shown by the Brundin group [34, 35], is elevated in blood after the TSST [181, 184] and an anger recall test [182], as well as in saliva after the exposure of police officers to a virtual gun confrontation [185]. Similarly, in saliva, IL-6 elevation occurs 10 and 20 min after the TSST, with a return to normal 60 min after completion of the TSST [186]. A meta-analysis found IL-6, but not other cytokines, to be significantly elevated in response to acute stress [187]. A review of the literature on the more convenient collection of inflammatory markers from saliva samples, rather than from blood [188], suggests that for the cytokines IL-1β, TNF-α and IL-6 saliva elevation in response to stress is highly apparent, significant and reliable. Experimentally in animals, stressors strongly upregulate tryptophan TDO and induce the production of kynurenines [189], partially through the activation of the HPA axis and the production of glucocorticoids [190]. More recently, stress also appears to produce kynurenines through IDO-1 and IDO-2 [191] activated by proinflammatory cytokines. Thus, stress itself can subjugate inflammation mechanisms and inflammation and kynurenine systems could mediate, in part, the effect of stress recognized by a stress diathesis model of suicide [52].

Conceptual Limitations

The immune system is a highly dynamic system, with proinflammatory, anti-inflammatory and regulatory processes alternating with potent reciprocal inhibitory connections. Changes in the levels of activity and thus exposure to the macroenvironment, changes in food intake and changes in metabolic/endocrine processes associated with the anguish that often builds up prior to a suicide attempt may influence the levels of inflammation, so that the observed inflammation might not be directly related to attempts but to behaviors preceding the attempts. The novel consistent evidence that acute stress upregulates certain proinflammatory cytokines raises the question of whether inflammation may be an epiphenomenon of suicidal behavior, as it may be a byproduct of the stress triggering suicidal behavior or of the presuicidal anguish.

Different compartments of the immune response – the innate and adaptive immunity, with myriads of cellular and molecular components – could have distinctly different associations with behavioral and psychological factors. It is very rare that research studies are able to analyze a large and comprehensive proportion of this complex interconnecting system. For instance, it may be difficult to tease apart the symptoms of suicidality from other aspects and symptoms of mental illness, in particular depression, that are highly intertwined with suicidal behavior. The majority of postmortem studies have this particular shortcoming and many of the clinical and epidemiological articles, even when attempting to control this by design, can only do this incompletely.

Measurements of immune mediators in plasma as well as ex vivo in cell culture supernatants do not reflect the exact changes that occur within the brain. Even in postmortem examinations as well as functional imaging studies, the findings of inflammation are quite brain region specific and it is not certain that the observed findings actually occur in a region of the brain that is of relevance to suicidal behavior.

Finally, within the brain the exact tissue specificity of the inflammatory findings is often not determined. For instance, the microglial, neuronal, astrocytic, or endothelial source is rarely dissected out using methods such as in situ hybridization. In the absence of tissue localization, it is possible that postmortem findings attributed to brain tissue (e.g. by PCR) could in fact originate in the vascular space-derived blood or perivascular structures surrounding the brain.

Conclusion

Much more remains to be done to better understand the association between the immune system and suicidal behavior. Study designs should attempt to match the complexity of the immune system and the interconnection between different components of the system and with other pathophysiological systems implicated in multiple risk factors for suicide. An emphasis on longitudinal designs, multiple complementary levels of inquiry and clinical trials with currently available pharmacological agents, many FDA approved for alternative indications, are expected to advance our knowledge as well as applications vertically. For instance, new interventions to be tested may include targeting microglial activation with minocycline, using specific cytokine blockers, addressing enzymes of kynurenine pathways, using antiparasitic treatment for preventing reactivation of *T. gondii*, or indicating the NMDA receptor antagonist ketamine more specifically to those with high kynurenine, high QUIN or high markers of inflammation. Ultimately, considering the magnitude of the problem and its resilience to usual approaches, no effort should be spared to find new angles for better prevention, prognosis and management of suicide risk.

Acknowledgments

Supported by the American Foundation for Suicide Prevention (Distinguished Investigator Award to TTP) and the Rocky Mountain MIRECC, Denver, Colo.

References

1 GBD 2013 Mortality and Causes of Death Collaborators: Global, regional, and national age-sex specific all-cause and cause-specific mortality for 240 causes of death, 1990–2013: a systematic analysis for the Global Burden of Disease Study 2013. Lancet, 2015; 385:117–171.
2 Krug EG, et al: The world report on violence and health. Lancet 2002;360:1083–1088.
3 Bertolote JM, Fleischmann A: Suicide and psychiatric diagnosis: a worldwide perspective. World Psychiatry 2002;1:181–185.
4 Mann JJ: Neurobiology of suicidal behaviour. Nat Rev Neurosci 2003;4:819–828.
5 Bach H, Arango V: Neuroanatomy of serotonergic abnormalities in suicide; in Dwivedi Y (ed): The Neurobiological Basis of Suicide, CRC Press, 2012.
6 Roy A, Sarchiopone M, Carli V: Gene-environment interaction and suicidal behavior. J Psychiatr Pract 2009;15:282–288.

7 Hawton K, van Heeringen K: Suicide. Lancet 2009;373:1372–1381.
8 Harris EC, Barraclough B: Suicide as an outcome for mental disorders. A meta-analysis. Br J Psychiatry 1997;170:205–228.
9 Dantzer R, et al: From inflammation to sickness and depression: when the immune system subjugates the brain. Nat Rev Neurosci 2008;9:46–56.
10 Borsini A, et al: The role of inflammatory cytokines as key modulators of neurogenesis. Trends Neurosci 2015;38:145–157.
11 Reichenberg A, et al: Cytokine-associated emotional and cognitive disturbances in humans. Arch Gen Psychiatry 2001;58:445–452.
12 Benros ME, et al: Autoimmune diseases and severe infections as risk factors for mood disorders: a nationwide study. JAMA Psychiatry 2013;70:812–820.
13 Maes M, et al: Depression's multiple comorbidities explained by (neuro) inflammatory and oxidative and nitrosative stress pathways. Neuroendocrinol Lett 2011;32:7–24.
14 Raison CL, Capuron L, Miller AH: Cytokines sing the blues: inflammation and the pathogenesis of depression. Trends Immunol 2006;27:24–31.
15 Raison CL, et al: Depression during pegylated interferon-α plus ribavirin therapy: prevalence and prediction. J Clin Psychiatry 2005;66:41.
16 Raison CL, et al: Activation of central nervous system inflammatory pathways by interferon-α: relationship to monoamines and depression. Biol Psychiatry 2009;65:296–303.
17 Raison CL, et al: CSF concentrations of brain tryptophan and kynurenines during immune stimulation with IFN-α: relationship to CNS immune responses and depression. Mol Psychiatry 2010;15:393–403.
18 Modabbernia A, et al: Cytokine alterations in bipolar disorder: a meta-analysis of 30 studies. Biol Psychiatry 2013;74:15–25.
19 Munkholm K, Vinberg M, Kessing LV: Cytokines in bipolar disorder: a systematic review and meta-analysis. J Affect Disord 2013;144:16–27.
20 Dargel AA, et al: C-reactive protein alterations in bipolar disorder: a meta-analysis. J Clin Psychiatry 2015;76:142–150.
21 Wium-Andersen MK, et al: Elevated C-reactive protein levels, psychological distress, and depression in 73,131 individuals. JAMA Psychiatry 2013;70:176–184.
22 Vogelzangs N, et al: Anxiety disorders and inflammation in a large adult cohort. Transl Psychiatry 2013;3:e249.
23 Rupprecht R, et al: Translocator protein (18 kDa) (TSPO) as a therapeutic target for neurological and psychiatric disorders. Nat Rev Drug Discov 2010;9:971–988.
24 Mizrahi R, et al: Translocator protein (18 kDa) polymorphism (rs6971) explains in-vivo brain binding affinity of the PET radioligand [^{18}F]-FEPPA. J Cereb Blood Flow Metab 2012;32:968–972.
25 Owen DR, et al: An 18-kDa translocator protein (TSPO) polymorphism explains differences in binding affinity of the PET radioligand PBR28. J Cereb Blood Flow Metab 2012;32:1–5.
26 Hannestad J, et al: The neuroinflammation marker translocator protein is not elevated in individuals with mild-to-moderate depression: A [^{11} C]PBR28 PET study. Brain Behav Immun 2013;33:131–138.
27 Setiawan E, et al: Role of translocator protein density, a marker of neuroinflammation, in the brain during major depressive episodes. JAMA Psychiatry 2015;72:268–275.
28 Dieperink E, et al: Suicidal ideation during interferon-α2b and ribavirin treatment of patients with chronic hepatitis C. Gen Hosp Psychiatry 2004;26:237–240.
29 Janssen HL, et al: Suicide associated with α-interferon therapy for chronic viral hepatitis. J Hepatol 1994;21:241–243.
30 Fragoso YD, et al: Severe depression, suicide attempts, and ideation during the use of interferon-β by patients with multiple sclerosis. Clin Neuropharmacol 2010;33:312–316.
31 Nassberger L, Traskman-Bendz L: Increased soluble interleukin-2 receptor concentrations in suicide attempters. Acta Psychiatr Scand 1993;88:48–52.
32 Tonelli LH, et al: Elevated cytokine expression in the orbitofrontal cortex of victims of suicide. Acta Psychiatr Scand 2008;117:198–206.
33 Steiner J, et al: Immunological aspects in the neurobiology of suicide: elevated microglial density in schizophrenia and depression is associated with suicide. J Psychiatr Res 2008;42:151–157.
34 Lindqvist D, et al: Interleukin-6 is elevated in the cerebrospinal fluid of suicide attempters and related to symptom severity. Biol Psychiatry 2009;66:287–292.
35 Janelidze S, et al: Cytokine levels in the blood may distinguish suicide attempters from depressed patients. Brain Behav Immun 2011;25:335–339.
36 Kim Y-K, et al: Differences in cytokines between non-suicidal patients and suicidal patients in major depression. Prog Neuropsychopharmacol Biol Psychiatry 2008;32:356–361.
37 Gabbay V, et al: A preliminary study of cytokines in suicidal and nonsuicidal adolescents with major depression. J Child Adolesc Psychopharmacol 2009;19:423–430.
38 Pandey GN, et al: Proinflammatory cytokines in the prefrontal cortex of teenage suicide victims. J Psychiatr Res 2012;46:57–63.
39 Falcone T, et al: Serum S100B: a potential biomarker for suicidality in adolescents? PLoS One 2010;5:e11089.

40 O'Donovan A, et al: Suicidal ideation is associated with elevated inflammation in patients with major depressive disorder. Depress Anxiety 2013;30:307–314.
41 Black C, Miller BJ: Meta-analysis of cytokines and chemokines in suicidality: distinguishing suicidal versus nonsuicidal patients. Biol Psychiatry 2015;78:28–31.
42 Serafini G, et al: The role of inflammatory cytokines in suicidal behavior: a systematic review. Eur Neuropsychopharmacol 2013;23:1672–1686.
43 Le-Niculescu H, et al: Discovery and validation of blood biomarkers for suicidality. Mol Psychiatry 2013;18:1249–1264.
44 Schéle E, et al: Interleukin-6 receptor α is co-localised with melanin-concentrating hormone in human and mouse hypothalamus. J Neuroendocrinol 2012;24:930–943.
45 Schobitz B, et al: Cellular localization of interleukin 6 mRNA and interleukin 6 receptor mRNA in rat brain. Eur J Neurosci 1993;5:1426–1435.
46 Ericsson A, et al: Type 1 interleukin-1 receptor in the rat brain: distribution, regulation, and relationship to sites of IL-1-induced cellular activation. J Comp Neurol 1995;361:681–698.
47 Tonelli LH, Postolache TT: Tumor necrosis factor-α, interleukin-1β, interleukin-6 and major histocompatibility complex molecules in the normal brain and after peripheral immune challenge. Neurol Res 2005;27:679–684.
48 Tonelli LH, Postolache TT, Sternberg EM: Inflammatory genes and neural activity: involvement of immune genes in synaptic function and behavior. Front Biosci 2005;10:675–680.
49 Kawasaki Y, et al: Cytokine mechanisms of central sensitization: distinct and overlapping role of interleukin-1β, interleukin-6, and tumor necrosis factor-α in regulating synaptic and neuronal activity in the superficial spinal cord. J Neurosci 2008;28:5189–5194.
50 Garcia-Oscos F, et al: The stress-induced cytokine interleukin-6 decreases the inhibition/excitation ratio in the rat temporal cortex via trans-signaling. Biol Psychiatry 2012;71:574–582.
51 Malkesman O, et al: Animal models of suicide-trait-related behaviors. Trends Pharmacol Sci 2009;30:165–173.
52 Mann JJ, et al: Candidate endophenotypes for genetic studies of suicidal behavior. Biol Psychiatry 2009;65:556–563.
53 Carroll JE, et al: Negative affective responses to a speech task predict changes in interleukin (IL)-6. Brain Behav Immun 2011;25:232–238.
54 Westling S, et al: Increased IL-1β reactivity upon a glucose challenge in patients with deliberate self-harm. Acta Psychiatr Scand 2011;124:301–306.
55 Bezemer G, et al: Psychiatric side effects and fluctuations in serotonergic parameters in the treatment of chronic hepatitis C infection. Neuropsychobiology 2012;65:126–132.
56 Lotrich FE, et al: Labile anger during interferon-α treatment is associated with a polymorphism in tumor necrosis factor-alpha. Clin Neuropharmacol 2010;33:191.
57 Hassanain M, et al: Interleukin-1β in the hypothalamus potentiates feline defensive rage: role of serotonin-2 receptors. Neuroscience 2003;120:227–233.
58 Bhatt S, et al: Role of IL-1β and 5-HT_2 receptors in midbrain periaqueductal gray (PAG) in potentiating defensive rage behavior in cat. Brain Behav Immun 2008;22:224–233.
59 Bhatt S, Siegel A: Potentiating role of interleukin 2 (IL-2) receptors in the midbrain periaqueductal gray (PAG) upon defensive rage behavior in the cat: role of neurokinin NK_1 receptors. Behav Brain Res 2006;167:251–260.
60 Patel A, Siegel A, Zalcman SS: Lack of aggression and anxiolytic-like behavior in TNF receptor (TNF-R1 and TNF-R2) deficient mice. Brain Behav Immun 2010;24:1276–1280.
61 Miller AH: Conceptual confluence: the kynurenine pathway as a common target for ketamine and the convergence of the inflammation and glutamate hypotheses of depression. Neuropsychopharmacology 2013;38:1607–1608.
62 Schwieler L, et al: Increased levels of IL-6 in the cerebrospinal fluid of patients with chronic schizophrenia-significance for activation of the kynurenine pathway. J Psychiatry Neurosci 2015;40:126–133.
63 Urata Y, et al: IL-1β increases expression of tryptophan 2, 3-dioxygenase and stimulates tryptophan catabolism in endometrioma stromal cells. Am J Reprod Immunol 2014;72:496–503.
64 Asberg M, Traskman L, Thoren P: 5-HIAA in the cerebrospinal fluid. A biochemical suicide predictor? Arch Gen Psychiatry 1976;33:1193–1197.
65 Schwarcz R, et al: Kynurenines in the mammalian brain: when physiology meets pathology. Nat Rev Neurosci 2012;13:465–477.
66 Leklem JE: Quantitative aspects of tryptophan metabolism in humans and other species: a review. Am J Clin Nutr 1971;24:659–672.
67 Stone TW: Neuropharmacology of quinolinic and kynurenic acids. Pharmacol Rev 1993;45:309–379.
68 de Carvalho LP, Bochet P, Rossier J: The endogenous agonist quinolinic acid and the nonendogenous homoquinolinic acid discriminate between NMDAR2 receptor subunits. Neurochem Int 1996;28:445–452.
69 Guillemin GJ: Quinolinic acid: neurotoxicity. FEBS J 2012;279:1355.

70 Erhardt S, Olsson SK, Engberg G: Pharmacological manipulation of kynurenic acid: potential in the treatment of psychiatric disorders. CNS Drugs 2009; 23:91–101.
71 Linderholm KR, et al: Increased levels of kynurenine and kynurenic acid in the CSF of patients with schizophrenia. Schizophr Bull 2012;38:426–432.
72 Sublette ME, et al: Plasma kynurenine levels are elevated in suicide attempters with major depressive disorder. Brain Behav Immun 2011;25:1272–1278.
73 Erhardt S, et al: Connecting inflammation with glutamate agonism in suicidality. Neuropsychopharmacology 2013;38:743–752.
74 Bay-Richter C, et al: A role for inflammatory metabolites as modulators of the glutamate N-methyl-D-aspartate receptor in depression and suicidality. Brain Behav Immun 2015;43:110–117.
75 Myint AM, et al: Kynurenine pathway in major depression: evidence of impaired neuroprotection. J Affect Disord 2007;98:143–151.
76 Savitz J, et al: Neuroprotective kynurenine metabolite indices are abnormally reduced and positively associated with hippocampal and amygdalar volume bipolar disorder. Psychoneuroendocrinology 2015; 52:200–211.
77 Savitz J, et al: Putative neuroprotective and neurotoxic kynurenine pathway metabolites are associated with hippocampal and amygdalar volumes in subjects with major depressive disorder. Neuropsychopharmacology 2015;40:463–471.
78 Monnerie H, Shashidhara S, Le Roux PD: Effect of excess extracellular glutamate on dendrite growth from cerebral cortical neurons at 3 days in vitro: involvement of NMDA receptors. J Neurosci Res 2003; 74:688–700.
79 Zunszain PA, et al: Interleukin-1β: a new regulator of the kynurenine pathway affecting human hippocampal neurogenesis. Neuropsychopharmacology 2012; 37:939–949.
80 van Heeringen K, et al: Is there a neuroanatomical basis of the vulnerability to suicidal behavior? A coordinate-based meta-analysis of structural and functional MRI studies. Front Hum Neurosci 2014;8:824.
81 Steiner J, et al: Severe depression is associated with increased microglial quinolinic acid in subregions of the anterior cingulate gyrus: evidence for an immune-modulated glutamatergic neurotransmission. J Neuroinflammation 2011;8:1–9.
82 Price RB, et al: Effects of intravenous ketamine on explicit and implicit measures of suicidality in treatment-resistant depression. Biol Psychiatry 2009;66: 522–526.
83 DiazGranados N, et al: Rapid resolution of suicidal ideation after a single infusion of an N-methyl-D-aspartate antagonist in patients with treatment-resistant major depressive disorder. J Clin Psychiatry 2010;71:1605–1611.
84 Ajioka I, et al: Differentiated horizontal interneurons clonally expand to form metastatic retinoblastoma in mice. Cell 2007;131:378–390.
85 Pappas G, Roussos N, Falagas ME: Toxoplasmosis snapshots: global status of Toxoplasma gondii seroprevalence and implications for pregnancy and congenital toxoplasmosis. Int J Parasitol 2009;39:1385–1394.
86 Dubey JP, Jones JL: *Toxoplasma gondii* infection in humans and animals in the United States. Int J Parasitol 2008;38:1257–1278.
87 Fekadu A, Shibre T, Cleare AJ: Toxoplasmosis as a cause for behaviour disorders – overview of evidence and mechanisms. Folia Parasitol (Praha) 2010;57: 105–113.
88 Flegr J, Kodym P, Tolarova V: Correlation of duration of latent *Toxoplasma gondii* infection with personality changes in women. Biol Psychol 2000;53: 57–68.
89 Lindova J, et al: Pattern of money allocation in experimental games supports the stress hypothesis of gender differences in *Toxoplasma gondii*-induced behavioural changes. Folia Parasitol 2010;57:136–142.
90 Havlicek J, et al: Decrease of psychomotor performance in subjects with latent 'asymptomatic' toxoplasmosis. Parasitology 2001;122:515–520.
91 Kocazeybek B, et al: Higher prevalence of toxoplasmosis in victims of traffic accidents suggests increased risk of traffic accident in *Toxoplasma*-infected inhabitants of Istanbul and its suburbs. Forensic Sci Int 2009;187:103–108.
92 Torrey EF, Bartko JJ, Yolken RH: *Toxoplasma gondii* and other risk factors for schizophrenia: an update. Schizophr Bull 2012;38:642–647.
93 Pearce BD, Kruszon-Moran D, Jones JL: The relationship between *Toxoplasma gondii* infection and mood disorders in the third National Health and Nutrition Survey. Biol Psychiatry 2012;72:290–295.
94 Hinze-Selch D, et al: The diagnosis of a personality disorder increases the likelihood for seropositivity to *Toxoplasma gondii* in psychiatric patients. Folia Parasitol (Praha) 2010;57:129–135.
95 Grant IH, et al: Toxoplasma gondii serology in HIV-infected patients: the development of central nervous system toxoplasmosis in AIDS. AIDS 1990;4: 519–521.
96 Meers S, et al: Myeloablative conditioning predisposes patients for *Toxoplasma gondii* reactivation after allogeneic stem cell transplantation. Clin Infect Dis 2010;50:1127–1134.
97 Vyas A, et al: Behavioral changes induced by *Toxoplasma* infection of rodents are highly specific to aversion of cat odors. Proc Natl Acad Sci U S A 2007; 104:6442–6447.
98 Afonso C, Paixao VB, Costa RM: Chronic *Toxoplasma* infection modifies the structure and the risk of host behavior. PLoS One 2012;7:e32489.

99 Gonzalez LE, et al: *Toxoplasma gondii* infection lower anxiety as measured in the plus-maze and social interaction tests in rats: a behavioral analysis. Behav Brain Res 2007;177:70–79.
100 Hay J, et al: The effect of congenital *Toxoplasma* infection on mouse activity and relative preference for exposed areas over a series of trials. Ann Trop Med Parasitol 1984;78:611–618.
101 Pepper M, Hunter CA: Innate recognition and the regulation of protective immunity to *Toxoplasma gondii*; in Ajioka AW, Soldati D (eds): *Toxoplasma*: Molecular and Cellular Biology. Norfolk, Horizon Bioscience, 2007, pp 111–126.
102 Arling TA, et al: Toxoplasma gondii antibody titers and history of suicide attempts in patients with recurrent mood disorders. J Nerv Ment Dis 2009;197: 905–908.
103 Okusaga O, et al: *Toxoplasma gondii* antibody titers and history of suicide attempts in patients with schizophrenia. Schizophr Res 2011;133:150–155.
104 Ling VJ, et al: *Toxoplasma gondii* seropositivity and suicide rates in women. J Nerv Ment Dis 2011;199: 440–444.
105 Pedersen MG, et al: *Toxoplasma gondii* infection and self-directed violence in mothers. Arch Gen Psychiatry 2012;69:1123–1130.
106 Zhang Y, et al: *Toxoplasma gondii* immunoglobulin G antibodies and nonfatal suicidal self-directed violence. J Clin Psychiatry 2012;73:1069–1076.
107 Yagmur F, et al: May *Toxoplasma gondii* increase suicide attempt – preliminary results in Turkish subjects? Forensic Sci Int 2010;199:15–17.
108 Samojlowicz D, Borowska-Solonynko A, Golab E: Prevalence of *Toxoplasma gondii* parasite infection among people who died due to sudden death in the capital city of Warsaw and its vicinity. Przegl Epidemiol 2013;67:29–33, 115–118.
109 Alvarado-Esquivel C, et al: *Toxoplasma gondii* infection and suicide attempts: a case-control study in psychiatric outpatients. J Nerv Ment Dis 2013; 201:948–952.
110 Cook TB, et al: 'Latent' infection with *Toxoplasma gondii*: association with trait aggression and impulsivity in healthy adults. J Psychiatr Res 2015;60:87–94.
111 Coccaro EF, et al: *Toxoplasma gondii* infection: relationship with other-directed and self-directed aggression in psychiatric subjects. J Clin Psychiatry, in press.
112 Patton JH, Stanford MS, Barratt ES: Factor structure of the Barratt impulsiveness scale. J Clin Psychol 1995;51:768–774.
113 Daubener W, MacKenzie CR: IFN-γ activated indoleamine 2,3-dioxygenase activity in human cells is an antiparasitic and an antibacterial effector mechanism. Adv Exp Med Biol 1999;467:517–524.
114 Notarangelo FM, et al: Evaluation of kynurenine pathway metabolism in *Toxoplasma gondii*-infected mice: implications for schizophrenia. Schizophr Res 2014;152:261–267.
115 Fallarino F, et al: The combined effects of tryptophan starvation and tryptophan catabolites down-regulate T cell receptor ζ-chain and induce a regulatory phenotype in naive T cells. J Immunol 2006; 176:6752–6761.
116 Edinger AL, Thompson CB: Antigen-presenting cells control T cell proliferation by regulating amino acid availability. Proc Natl Acad Sci U S A 2002; 99:1107–1109.
117 Munn DH, et al: Inhibition of T cell proliferation by macrophage tryptophan catabolism. J Exp Med 1999;189:1363–1372.
118 Mellor AL, et al: Cutting edge: induced indoleamine 2,3-dioxygenase expression in dendritic cell subsets suppresses T cell clonal expansion. J Immunol 2003;171:1652–1655.
119 Bauer TM, et al: Studying the immunosuppressive role of indoleamine 2,3-dioxygenase: tryptophan metabolites suppress rat allogeneic T-cell responses in vitro and in vivo. Transpl Int 2005;18:95–100.
120 Frumento G, et al: Tryptophan-derived catabolites are responsible for inhibition of T and natural killer cell proliferation induced by indoleamine 2,3-dioxygenase. J Exp Med 2002;196:459–468.
121 Nguyen NT, et al: Aryl hydrocarbon receptor negatively regulates dendritic cell immunogenicity via a kynurenine-dependent mechanism. Proc Natl Acad Sci U S A 2010;107:19961–19966.
122 Mezrich JD, et al: An interaction between kynurenine and the aryl hydrocarbon receptor can generate regulatory T cells. J Immunol 2010;185:3190–3198.
123 Prendergast GC, et al: Indoleamine 2,3-dioxygenase pathways of pathogenic inflammation and immune escape in cancer. Cancer Immunol Immunother 2014;63:721–735.
124 Moretti S, et al: Indoleamine 2,3-dioxygenase 1 (IDO1) is up-regulated in thyroid carcinoma and drives the development of an immunosuppressant tumor microenvironment. J Clin Endocrinol Metab 2014;99:E832–E840.
125 Opitz CA, et al: An endogenous tumour-promoting ligand of the human aryl hydrocarbon receptor. Nature 2011;478:197–203.
126 Gaskell EA, et al: A unique dual activity amino acid hydroxylase in *Toxoplasma gondii*. PLoS One 2009; 4:e4801.
127 Chew KSY, McCleary R: The spring peak in suicides: a cross-national analysis. Soc Sci Med 1995; 40:223–230.
128 Christodoulou C, et al: Suicide and seasonality. Acta Psychiatr Scand 2012;125:127–146.

129 Maes M, et al: Seasonality in severity of depression: relationships to suicide and homicide occurrence. Acta Psychiatr Scand 1993;88:156–161.
130 Petridou E, et al: A role of sunshine in the triggering of suicide. Epidemiology 2002;13:106–109.
131 Postolache TT, et al: Seasonal spring peaks of suicide in victims with and without prior history of hospitalization for mood disorders. J Affect Disord 2010;121:88–93.
132 Woo JM, Okusaga O, Postolache TT: Seasonality of suicidal behavior. Int J Environ Res Public Health 2012;9:531–547.
133 Yip P, Chao A, Chiu C: Seasonal variation in suicides: diminished or vanished experience from England and Wales, 1982–1996. Br J Psychiatry 2000;177:366–369.
134 Okusaga O, et al: Association of seropositivity for influenza and coronaviruses with history of mood disorders and suicide attempts. J Affect Disord 2011;130:220–225.
135 Postolache TT, et al: Tree pollen peaks are associated with increased nonviolent suicide in women. Mol Psychiatry 2005;10:232–235.
136 Woo JM, et al: Pollen counts and suicide rates. Association not replicated. Acta Psychiatr Scand 2012;125:168–175.
137 Qin P, et al: Suicide risk in relation to air pollen counts: a study based on data from Danish registers. BMJ Open 2013;3:e002462.
138 Tonelli LH, et al: Allergic rhinitis induces anxiety-like behavior and altered social interaction in rodents. Brain Behav Immun 2009;23:784–793.
139 Tonelli LH, et al: Acute stress promotes aggressive-like behavior in rats made allergic to tree pollen. Int J Child Health Hum Dev 2008;1:305–312.
140 Woo JM, et al: Suicide and prescription rates of intranasal corticosteroids and nonsedating antihistamines for allergic rhinitis: an ecological study. J Clin Psychiatry 2011;72:1423–1428.
141 Manalai P, et al: Pollen-specific immunoglobulin E positivity is associated with worsening of depression scores in bipolar disorder patients during high pollen season. Bipolar Disord 2012;14:90–98.
142 Goodwin RD: Asthma and suicide: current knowledge and future directions. Curr Psychiatry Rep 2012;14:30–35.
143 Qin P, et al: Allergy is associated with suicide completion with a possible mediating role of mood disorder – a population-based study. Allergy 2011;66: 658–664.
144 Kim C, et al: Ambient particulate matter as a risk factor for suicide. Am J Psychiatry 2010;167:1100–1107.
145 Tonelli LH, Holmes A, Postolache TT: Intranasal immune challenge induces sex-dependent depressive-like behavior and cytokine expression in the brain. Neuropsychopharmacology 2008;33:1038–1048.
146 Postolache TT, Komarow H, Tonelli LH: Allergy: a risk factor for suicide? Curr Treat Options Neurol 2008;10:363–376.
147 Fang BJ, et al: Disturbed sleep: linking allergic rhinitis, mood and suicidal behavior. Front Biosci (Schol Ed) 2010;2:30–46.
148 Holick MF: Vitamin D deficiency. New Engl J Med 2007;357:266–281.
149 Tangpricha V, et al: Vitamin D insufficiency among free-living healthy young adults. Am J Med 2002; 112:659–662.
150 Eyles DW, et al: Distribution of the vitamin D receptor and 1α-hydroxylase in human brain. J Chem Neuroanat 2005;29:21–30.
151 De Abreu DAF, Eyles D, Feron F: Vitamin D, a neuro-immunomodulator: implications for neurodegenerative and autoimmune diseases. Psychoneuroendocrinology 2009;34:S265–S277.
152 Lemire JM, et al: 1 alpha,25-dihydroxyvitamin D3 suppresses proliferation and immunoglobulin production by normal human peripheral blood mononuclear cells. J Clin Invest 1984;74:657.
153 Szodoray P, et al: The complex role of vitamin D in autoimmune diseases. Scand J Immunol 2008;68: 261–269.
154 Liu PT, et al: Toll-like receptor triggering of a vitamin D-mediated human antimicrobial response. Science 2006;311:1770–1773.
155 Cannell JJ, et al: Epidemic influenza and vitamin D. Epidemiol Infect 2006;134:1129–1140.
156 Hewison M: Vitamin D and the immune system: new perspectives on an old theme. Endocrinol Metab Clin North Am 2010;39:365–379.
157 Correale J, Ysrraelit MC, Gaitán MI: Immunomodulatory effects of vitamin D in multiple sclerosis. Brain 2009;132(pt 59):1146–1160.
158 Gorman S, et al: Topically applied 1,25-dihydroxyvitamin D3 enhances the suppressive activity of CD4+ CD25+ cells in the draining lymph nodes. J Immunol 2007;179:6273–6283.
159 Tariq MM, et al: Vitamin D: a potential role in reducing suicide risk? Int J Adolesc Med Health 2011; 23:157–165.
160 Umhau JC, et al: Low vitamin D status and suicide: a case-control study of active duty military service members. PLoS One 2013;8:e51543.
161 Grudet C, et al: Suicidal patients are deficient in vitamin D, associated with a pro-inflammatory status in the blood. Psychoneuroendocrinology 2014;50: 210–219.
162 Meszaros ZS, Perl A, Faraone SV: Psychiatric symptoms in systemic lupus erythematosus: a systematic review. J Clin Psychiatry 2012;73:993–1001.
163 Chwastiak L, et al: Depressive symptoms and severity of illness in multiple sclerosis: epidemiologic study of a large community sample. Am J Psychiatry 2002;159:1862–1868.

164 Lauvsnes MB, Omdal R: Systemic lupus erythematosus, the brain, and anti-NR2 antibodies. J Neurol 2012;259:622–629.
165 Fredrikson S, et al: Elevated suicide risk among patients with multiple sclerosis in Sweden. Neuroepidemiology 2002;22:146–152.
166 Brønnum-Hansen H, et al: Suicide among Danes with multiple sclerosis. J Neurol Neurosurg Psychiatry 2005;76:1457–1459.
167 Ludvigsson JF, et al: Increased suicide risk in coeliac disease – a Swedish nationwide cohort study. Dig Liver Dis 2011;43:616–622.
168 Okusaga O, et al: Elevated gliadin antibody levels in individuals with schizophrenia. World J Biol Psychiatry 2013;14:509–515.
169 Fazel S, et al: Suicide, fatal injuries, and other causes of premature mortality in patients with traumatic brain injury: a 41-year Swedish population study. JAMA Psychiatry 2014;71:326–333.
170 Town T, Nikolic V, Tan J: The microglial "activation" continuum: from innate to adaptive responses. J Neuroinflammation 2005;2:24.
171 Herber DL, et al: Diverse microglial responses after intrahippocampal administration of lipopolysaccharide. Glia 2006;53:382–391.
172 Lehnardt S: Innate immunity and neuroinflammation in the CNS: the role of microglia in Toll-like receptor-mediated neuronal injury. Glia 2010;58: 253–263.
173 Beattie MS, Ferguson AR, Bresnahan JC: AMPA-receptor trafficking and injury-induced cell death. Eur J Neurosci 2010;32:290–297.
174 Rodgers KM, et al: The cortical innate immune response increases local neuronal excitability leading to seizures. Brain 2009;132:2478–2486.
175 Juengst SB, et al: Exploratory associations with tumor necrosis factor-α, disinhibition and suicidal endorsement after traumatic brain injury. Brain Behav Immun 2014;41:134–143.
176 Mackay GM, et al: Tryptophan metabolism and oxidative stress in patients with chronic brain injury. Eur J Neurol 2006;13:30–42.
177 Mastrolonardo M, et al: Effect of psychological stress on salivary interleukin-1β in psoriasis. Arch Med Res 2007;38:206–211.
178 Mahmood A, Ibrahim L: Effect of the examination stress on periodontal health status and salivary IL-1B among Iraqi dental students. J Baghdad Coll Dent 2013;24:72–78.
179 Kirschbaum C, Pirke KM, Hellhammer DH: The 'Trier Social Stress Test' – a tool for investigating psychobiological stress responses in a laboratory setting. Neuropsychobiology 1993;28:76–81.
180 Altemus M, et al: Stress-induced changes in skin barrier function in healthy women. J Invest Dermatol 2001;117:309–317.
181 Bower JE, et al: Inflammatory responses to psychological stress in fatigued breast cancer survivors: relationship to glucocorticoids. Brain Behav Immun 2007;21:251–258.
182 Suarez EC, et al: Increases in stimulated secretion of proinflammatory cytokines by blood monocytes following arousal of negative affect: the role of insulin resistance as moderator. Brain Behav Immun 2006;20:331–338.
183 Heesen C, et al: Endocrine and cytokine responses to acute psychological stress in multiple sclerosis. Brain Behav Immun 2002;16:282–287.
184 Rohleder N, et al: Impact of oral contraceptive use on glucocorticoid sensitivity of pro-inflammatory cytokine production after psychosocial stress. Psychoneuroendocrinology 2003;28:261–273.
185 Groer M, et al: Salivary measures of stress and immunity in police officers engaged in simulated critical incident scenarios. J Occup Environ Med 2010; 52:595–602.
186 Izawa S, et al: An increase in salivary interleukin-6 level following acute psychosocial stress and its biological correlates in healthy young adults. Biol Psychol 2013;94:249–254.
187 Steptoe A, Hamer M, Chida Y: The effects of acute psychological stress on circulating inflammatory factors in humans: a review and meta-analysis. Brain Behav Immun 2007;21:901–912.
188 Slavish DC, et al: Salivary markers of inflammation in response to acute stress. Brain Behav Immun 2015;44:253–269.
189 Miura H, et al: Changes in brain tryptophan metabolism elicited by ageing, social environment, and psychological stress in mice. Stress 2008;11: 160–169.
190 Salter M, Pogson CI: The role of tryptophan 2,3-dioxygenase in the hormonal control of tryptophan metabolism in isolated rat liver cells. Effects of glucocorticoids and experimental diabetes. Biochem J 1985;229:499–504.
191 Kiank C, et al: Psychological stress-induced, IDO-1-dependent tryptophan catabolism: implications on immunosuppression in mice and humans. PLoS One 2010;5:e11825.

Teodor T. Postolache, MD
Department of Psychiatry, University of Maryland-Baltimore School of Medicine
685 W. Baltimore Street, Room 930
Baltimore, MD 21201 (USA)
E-Mail tpostola@psych.umaryland.edu

Kaschka WP, Rujescu D (eds): Biological Aspects of Suicidal Behavior.
Adv Biol Psychiatry. Basel, Karger, 2016, vol 30, pp 145–160 (DOI: 10.1159/000434747)

The Contributions of Lithium and Clozapine for the Prophylaxis and Treatment of Suicidal Behavior

Bruno Müller-Oerlinghausen[a] · Ute Lewitzka[b]

[a]Charité Universitäts-Medizin Berlin and Freie Universität Berlin, Berlin, and [b]Department of Psychiatry and Psychotherapy, University Hospital Carl Gustav Carus, Technische Universität Dresden, Dresden, Germany

Abstract

The fact that various drugs with different mechanisms of action can induce suicidality even in people who never had suicidal ideation before suggests that the neurobiological correlates of suicidal ideation and behavior are complex and not very well understood. Lithium and clozapine are unique substances since they are the only psychotropic compounds for which evidence of an antisuicidal effect exists so far. In this chapter the scientific proof for such effect will be unfolded in a narrative review. Particularly for lithium salts, this effect has been documented since the 90s in a large number of studies with quite different methodological approaches by various international research groups. It could be shown beyond any doubt that the 2- to 3-times elevated standardized mortality of patients with affective disorders can be reduced by a well-monitored lithium prophylaxis to the level of the general population. Various studies suggest that other 'mood stabilizers' do not possess this property, at least not to the same extent. Some authors based on their studies have concluded that this lithium effect might be specific, i.e. independent of lithium's episode-preventing activity. Clozapine possesses antisuicidal and, similar to lithium, also antiaggressive effects and efficacy in schizophrenic patients, although the evidence is not as strong as with lithium, considering the smaller number of large studies. Clozapine also counteracts aggressive and self-mutilating behavior in patients with personality disorders. Possible neurobiological mechanisms underlying these unique effects of lithium and clozapine are discussed at the end of the chapter, for example changes in postsynaptic 5-HT_{1A} receptor activity might be a link between certain clinical effects of antidepressants, lithium and clozapine.

Various chapters of this book provide ample evidence that suicidal behavior can be caused by or rather is associated with not only psychosocial, spiritual, emotional, or cognitive but also biological factors per se. This becomes evident also from the longstanding observation that a large variety of drugs can induce depressive states, suicidal ideation and suicidal behavior. Among them we find pharmacologically quite different compounds such as, for example, interferon-α, mefloquine, isotretinoin, finasteride, fluoroquinolones, and quite surprisingly, even antidepressants, particularly SSRIs [1–4]. The underlying mechanisms are mostly unclear. For example, a potential negative influence on precursors of the serotonin metabolism has been discussed for interferon-α [5]. Glutamatergic and GABAergic mechanisms might play a role in the suicidogenic effects of finasteride. On a behavioral level, excitatory, anxiety-inducing effects have been made responsible for the suicide-provoking effects of SSRIs. Whether such effects would also be responsible for antidepressant-induced emergent suicidal ideation in patients who never before had shown any suicidal ideation or behavior, however, is unclear. Fortunately, only a small number of patients will develop suicidality triggered by antidepressants; children and adolescents appear to be at special risk. This implies that special unknown resilience factors preventing this side effect obviously must exist and that the mental and biological factors defining an individual proneness to suicidal thoughts and behavior might be different in adolescents and adults. Interestingly, some recent findings suggest a genetic predisposition for the occurrence of this occasionally fatal adverse drug reaction [6].

In contrast to the great number of compounds possessing depressogenic/suicidogenic properties, pharmaceutical agents that could effectively counteract suicidality or diminish an increased long-term risk of committing suicide are surprisingly rare. Only two compounds exist for which robust or at least satisfactory evidence of an antisuicidal efficacy exists in patients with affective disorders or schizophrenia – lithium salts and clozapine. Lithium's very convincingly documented antisuicidal effects have become a strong argument for its high ranking in recent guidelines having classified lithium as a first-choice agent for the long-term treatment of patients with bipolar disorders (e.g. Deutsche Gesellschaft für Bipolare Störungen/Deutsche Gesellschaft für Psychiatrie, Psychotherapie und Nervenheilkunde, DGBS/DGPPN).

It appears particularly puzzling that antidepressants do not possess a specific antisuicidal effect. Clearly, in a case where suicidal ideation is embedded in an acute depressive state, an improvement of depression would also result in a reduction of the frequency and impact of suicidal thoughts. However, claims that antidepressants could reduce the inherent suicide risk in patients with affective disorders are not in accordance with the overall scientific evidence [7]. Thus, none of 6 meta-analyses comprising between 20,000 and 90,000 patients from published RCTs found a significant reduction of suicidal acts in the antidepressant versus the placebo groups. In the meta-analysis of Fergusson et al. [8], the rate of suicides and suicide attempts was even higher in the SSRI group compared to placebo. A recent reanalysis by Gibbons et al. [9] referring only to fluoxetine and venlafaxine also clearly shows that in adults the development of suicidal acts and overall suicidal ideation over time does not differ between the antidepressant and the placebo group.

Lithium

In the following we do not intend to provide the reader with a comprehensive overview on the existing studies in this area [10]. Rather, we are going to document the existence of the antisuicidal effects of lithium and clozapine, referring to a selection of representative and valid studies and also reviews in this area. This will also include a discussion of the data suggesting antisuicidal/antiaggressive efficacy of lithium as a trace element in large epidemiological studies. We shall outline in short the history and development of international research on the suicide-preventive effect of lithium. We then discuss the potential specificity of the antisuicidal effect, focusing on the questions: (1) whether the suicide- and mortality-reducing effect of lithium is shared by other psychotropics including mood stabilizers and (2) whether this effect might be independent of the episode-suppressing effect.

Can Adequate Lithium Prophylaxis Change the Suicide Risk and Mortality of Patients with Affective Disorders?

Patients with affective disorders exhibit a 2- to 3-times increased mortality compared to the general population [11, 12]. This excess mortality is caused primarily by the possibly 30- to 70-fold higher suicide-related mortality [13] – which is particularly high in patients with a history of suicide attempt [14, 15]. The meta-analysis by Guze and Robins [16] calculated the lifetime suicide risk as 15% for affective disorders, whereas 20 years later Goodwin and Jamison [17] – based on more recent literature – reported an overall risk of 19%. According to the WHO [18] the lifetime risk ranges between 6 and 15%. According to a recent review the life-time risk of suicide in patients with mood disorders is 5–6%, with possibly a higher risk in patients with bipolar disorders [19].

As reported by Harris and Barraclough [20], the suicide-related standardized mortality ratio (SMR) is 21.24 in major depression and 11.73 in bipolar disorder, with, however, large confidence intervals [21].

The intriguing question of whether long-term medication with lithium salts can improve the course of the manic depressive illness or of affective disorders in terms of suicide prevention has been given little attention up to the 80s (table 1).

Barraclough [22] was one of the first investigators postulating a potential association between lithium long-term medication and suicide prevention. Based on a detailed analysis of the charts of 100 suicide victims he concluded that about 20% of the suicides could have been prevented by adequate lithium medication. The first systematic retrospective study demonstrating a highly significant reduction of suicide attempts in a sample of 64 high-risk patients (46 bipolar and 11 schizoaffective) during long-term lithium treatment was published by Müller-Oerlinghausen et al. [23]. The authors emphasized that suicides and suicide attempts occurred nearly

Table 1. Antisuicidal effect of lithium: history

Anecdotal reports and findings from follow-ups in the 70s and 80s on possible reduction of suicidal behavior in lithium-treated patients	Barraclough [22], 1972 and others
First systematic follow-up studies of high-risk patients during long-term lithium treatment	
Berlin study: 2 suicides, 4 suicide attempts in 55 patients with regular lithium treatment; 4 suicides, 7 suicide attempts in 13 patients having discontinued lithium	Müller-Oerlinghausen et al. [23], 1992
Dresden study: 6 suicide attempts in 36 patients on lithium; 3 suicides, 36 suicide attempts in 36 patients off lithium	Felber and Kyber [24], 1994
Mortality studies	
First Berlin studies on general mortality-reducing effects of lithium	Ahrens and Müller-Oerlinghausen [26], 1990
Coppen shows reduced mortality in mostly unipolar patients on lithium	Coppen et al. [25], 1991
The IGSLI studies on mortality (MORTA I-IV) First systematic multicenter analysis of about 6,000 patient years	Müller-Oerlinghausen et al. [28, 29], 1992, 1994; Ahrens et al. [21], 1995; Ahrens and Müller-Oerlinghausen [26], 1990
Further studies	
The MAP study, randomized, prospective, treatment time 2.5 years, n = 285. No suicidal acts on lithium, 9 suicidal acts on carbamazepine	Thies-Flechtner et al. [45], 1996; Greil et al. [46], 1997
2 large Swedish studies and 1 Sardinian study confirm the IGSLI findings	Kallner et al. [34], 2000
Review of the existing data: risk of suicidal acts 7-8 times higher in bipolar patients off lithium	Tondo et al. [39], 1997

exclusively in a group of 13 patients who had taken lithium irregularly or had stopped the medication.

Felber and Kyber [24] in Dresden analyzed suicide attempts during accumulated periods on and off lithium and had very similar findings – 90% of the suicide attempts occurred in the off-lithium period.

Several studies on the mortality of affective disorders during lithium long-term treatment by Coppen et al. [25] and Ahrens and Müller-Oerlinghausen [26] demonstrated that the SMR of patients with affective disorders during adequate lithium medication is normalized down to the level of the general population. Coppen [27] reviewed the studies existing in the mid-90s on the suicide rates in patients on versus off lithium and concluded that adequate lithium medication reduces suicide-related mortality by 82%.

The IGSLI Studies

In the main study of IGSLI (International Group for The Study of Lithium-Treated Patients) well-documented data on the course of illness of 827 patients with affective disorders from specialized lithium clinics in Austria, Canada, Denmark, and Germany who had been treated with lithium for at least 6 months were evaluated – 55% of the patients were bipolar, 25% unipolar, 2% unipolar-manic, 16% schizoaffective, and 2% had other diagnoses [21, 28]. At the onset of the lithium prophylaxis the patients were on average 41 years old. The mean duration of lithium treatment was 81 months (6–21 years), equaling 5,600 patient-years.

The ratio of 44 observed and 38 expected cases of death is not statistically different from 1.0, which is the mortality of the general population. Thus, the expected 2- to 3-fold excess mortality in patients with affective disorders (see above) did not exist in this lithium-treated patient sample. Bipolar patients do not differ essentially from other diagnostic groups in this respect.

Although the specific suicide-related SMR was still higher than in the general population it could clearly be shown that it was definitely lower in all diagnostic groups compared to what could be expected in untreated patient samples.

It has been argued on various occasions that patients accepting a lithium prophylaxis might generally benefit from a better prognosis. In this case the specific patient selection would have been primarily responsible for the normalization of the SMR. To study this issue, in a successive analysis of 270 German and Danish patients from the original IGSLI sample the initial SMR was compared to the SMR after treatment of more than 1 year [29]. During the first year the overall mortality was increased 2-fold and the suicide-related mortality 17-fold compared to the general population. The SMR normalized after the first year of treatment, indicating that patients for whom lithium prophylaxis is indicated are in fact patients with a high risk of suicide.

Confirmatory data came from Italy when Bocchetta et al. [30] demonstrated a 6-fold decreased incidence of suicide attempts in 100 carefully monitored and documented lithium patients. During the observational period of approximately 10 years, 10 suicides occurred in this cohort – 9 of them in patients having discontinued their lithium medication. A year later a well-known research group in Boston (USA) also showed in a cohort of 300 bipolar patients that the incidence of suicide increased 20-fold in the first year after ending a foregoing lithium medication [31].

Further Studies on Mortality

As mentioned above it was also argued that the reduction of mortality might essentially be due to the optimal care and attention patients receive in specialized lithium clinics. In this context 2 Swedish studies are of particular interest. In an open-field setting Nilsson [32] could not observe a full normalization of the SMR. However, as in other studies, Schou [33] found a rise of the SMR up to the expected level in untreated affective disorders after the discontinuation of lithium.

Kallner et al. [34] analyzed a mixed sample of 497 Swedish patients including 405 bipolar patients treated with lithium during an observation period of 30 years. The patients were divided into three groups according to the regularity of attending the study clinic. Among the bipolar patients the suicide rate was in excess in all three groups. However, the suicide rate was increased by 80% when patients stopped taking lithium. This study deserves special attention because on one side it generally confirms the findings by the IGSLI and by Nilsson but it also suggests that the suicide-preventing effect of lithium might be more marked in patients being taken care of in specialized lithium clinics. The suicide-related SMR in patients on lithium was 14.0 when they had regular visits to the clinic and 21.4 when treated elsewhere. This difference could possibly be explained by the generally higher quality of the treatment regimens and by the closer monitoring of the patients.

In 2005 Angst et al. [35] published a study of 406 patients with affective disorders who had been followed up over 40 years (the so-called Zurich cohort). The patients treated with lithium had a lower than expected mortality rate which was not different from the mortality rate of the general population.

There are very few studies apparently contradicting the findings of IGSLI. Thus, Vestergaard and Aagaard [36] and Brodersen et al. [37] were not able to demonstrate reduced mortality in cohorts of lithium-treated manic-depressive patients. However, the average duration of the lithium treatment was less than in the IGSLI study and control of compliance might not have been sufficient – one third of the deaths that occurred in their study took place after patients discontinued lithium. Another negative though very small study was published by Coryell et al. [38].

Reviews and Meta-Analyses

The first meta-analysis on about 17,000 bipolar patients was published by the Boston group in 1997 [39]. It demonstrated an 8.6-fold higher mortality from suicide in patients treated without lithium than in patients during lithium long-term treatment.

Cipriani et al. [40] from Oxford meta-analyzed RCTs on the episode-preventive efficacy of lithium and found a very clear and highly significant reduction of suicidal acts and mortality for lithium compared to either placebo or any other psychotropics, including antidepressants. An updated version of this analysis was published by the same authors in 2013 [41]. The meta-analysis by Baldessarini et al. [42] published in 2006 referred to 33,000 patients and 45 studies and also proved that lithium-treated patients had a 5-fold decreased risk for suicidal acts and reduced overall mortality compared to patients having been given other medication.

An RCT to Explore the Suicide-Protective Effect of Lithium

There are many methodological obstacles to perform controlled prospective trials in the area of suicidology. First, the study protocol will usually exclude patients with suicidal tendencies from drug trials. Second, from an ethical point of view, placebo-controlled studies with suicide or suicide attempt as primary outcome will hardly be acceptable. Third – since suicide is fortunately a relatively rare event – large patient numbers would be needed to reach sufficient statistical power, resulting in a nearly unsolvable ethical dilemma. Nevertheless, an independently sponsored RCT from Germany, which due to the above-mentioned and additional methodological difficulties could not be performed in full concordance with the requirements of the power calculation, had an interesting and confirmatory result. Within the treatment period of 1 year no suicides occurred in the lithium group (n = 84), whereas 3 suicides occurred in the placebo group (n = 84) [43]. Interestingly, a post hoc analysis did not show a suicide-protective effect in those patients of the study who had also been given a diagnosis of personality disorder [44].

Is the Anti-Suicidal and Mortality-Reducing Effect of Lithium Specific?

In view of these rather robust and consistent findings the intriguing question arises whether the suicide-preventive effect of lithium should be considered a 'specific' effect – and what could be the underlying mechanism?

For the sake of clarity we may subdivide the issue of potential specificity into two questions, as follows:

(1) Is this effect specific for lithium salts – in other words, is it not shared by other drugs such as other mood stabilizers or antidepressants?

(2) Is this effect strictly related to the episode-preventive effect of lithium prophylaxis or might it act independently?

The question of whether the antisuicidal effect is shared by other psychotropic agents was addressed in the German multicenter MAP study – a prospective RCT with a treatment time of 2.5 years. In total, 146 bipolar and schizoaffective patients were randomized on lithium and 139 on carbamazepine. No suicidal act was observed in the lithium group. However, 4 suicides and 5 suicide attempts occurred in the carbamazepine group – a statistically significant difference [45–47].

A study by Goodwin et al. [48] comparing the suicide risk in lithium- versus valproate-treated patients has found much attention in the USA. The authors conducted a retrospective cohort study on two large integrated health plans in California and Washington. In this follow-up of more than 20,000 patients who received lithium, carbamazepine or valproate between 1994 and 2001 the adjusted suicide risk was 2.7 times (95% CI 1.1–6.3; p = 0.03) higher in the valproate-treated patients compared to the lithium-treated patients. Hazard ratios for suicide attempts amounted to 1.7–1.8. In addition, the carbamazepine-treated patients had a significantly higher risk of suicide attempts leading to hospitalization in comparison to patients having been prescribed lithium at least once during the observation period.

Collins and McFarland [49] investigated 12,626 Medicaid-insured patients and demonstrated that lithium-treated bipolar patients had the lowest number of suicide attempts compared to those having been prescribed other mood stabilizers.

Oquendo et al. [50] observed the effect of lithium compared to valproate in the prevention of suicidal behavior in patients with bipolar disorder over a period of 2.5 years. During that randomized clinical trial no suicides occurred within the whole study sample. Overall, 6 suicide attempts were registered in the lithium group (n = 49) and 8 in the valproate group (n = 49). Unfortunately, due to a high attrition rate, the study lost considerable statistical power. In this context it might also be worth mentioning that in the RCT by Lauterbach et al. [43] only the incidence of suicides, but not of suicide attempts, differed between the lithium and the placebo group.

In a large study by Weisler et al. [51] comparing the effect of prolonged quetiapine medication versus switching to placebo or lithium for maintenance treatment in 2,438 bipolar I patients, only 1 suicidal/accidental gunshot wound was observed during the open-label treatment with quetiapine. During the randomized phase only a low and similar overall incidence of suicidal behavior/ideation was observed in the quetiapine (n = 3), lithium (n = 3) and placebo (n = 8) groups.

Khan et al. [52] published a study primarily designed to investigate whether the antisuicidal effects of lithium can be prospectively evaluated using lithium as an augmenting agent to antidepressants. A subgroup of the patients assigned to citalopram and lithium achieved therapeutic serum levels and had significantly higher S-STS (Sheehan Suicidality Tracking Scale) remission rates compared to patients assigned to citalopram or placebo alone. They debated that lithium when used in therapeutic doses may augment a direct therapeutic effect of citalopram on suicidal thoughts and behavior.

Taken together, some studies suggest that a few nonlithium compounds might protect patients with mood disorders against suicidal acts to some extent. Such potential and possibly only modest effects, however, can hardly be documented in a study cohort showing only a low suicide risk.

What Could Be the Mechanism of This Suicide-Preventive Effect?

While it was postulated by Baldessarini et al. [53] that the reduction of the suicide risk by lithium prophylaxis is primarily caused by its depression-preventive effect, the hypothesis of the Berlin group from the very beginning has always been that lithium differs from other mood stabilizers and also from most antidepressants by its very marked serotonin agonistic effects which are related predominantly to its presynaptic functions [54, 55]. It appears to be at least an attractive speculation that this serotoninergic action of lithium, possibly in connection with other effects, is related to its very well-established antiaggressive effects in animals as well as humans [56, 57] but also to its antisuicidal effects. In one of the rare animal studies focusing on potential neurobiological underpinnings of the clinical effects of lithium, Ohmura et al. [58] investigated whether major mood-stabilizing drugs used for the treatment of bipolar disorder could suppress impulsive-like action in the three-choice serial reaction time task in rats. The authors debated that lithium, but not valproate or carbamazepine, may suppress impulsive behavior and thereby decrease the risk of suicide. Shock-induced aggression in mice is also attenuated by lithium, as shown by Kovacsics and Gould [59]. Overall, neurobiological research has focused on lithium's influence on neurotransmitters such as serotonin, noradrenalin and dopamine, the cortisol stress hormone system, the γ-aminobutyric-acid, second-messenger systems such as inositol metabolism, glycogen synthase kinase 3, and more. The most favored hypothesis is that lithium leads to a decrease of impulsivity and aggression via several influences within the nerve cell [57, 60]. The neurobiological research on suicide at present points to an important influence of overactivity of the corticotropin-releasing hormone, as well as of the noradrenergic system, and a dysfunction of the serotonergic system [61, 62]. There could be a link between these dysfunctions and microglial hyperactivity. Thus, quinolinic acid derived from tryptophan could lead to a lowered cerebral level of tryptophan and serotonin [63]. Could it be that lithium by its serotonin agonistic properties counteracts this deficiency on the neurotransmitter level? We may also approach the problem from another side, i.e. considering the endophenotype of a suicidal individual [64]. Some findings suggest that suicidal behavior might be seen as a particular, possibly anger-related form of affective dysregulation that is also associated with disturbance of the serotonin (5-HT) system and, thus, as a more or less independent nosological entity. Thus, according to data from the WHO study from the year 2000 the prevalence of suicidal ideation and behavior is not fully related to the existence of ICD psychiatric diagnoses but it occurs frequently in asymptomatic individuals and in subjects with subthreshold disorders [65]. Many such people are characterized by symptoms of overt or suppressed anger [66] which van Praag [67] considers as one of the core constituents of the stress syndrome, together with anxiety. He postulated that in certain types of depression – characterized by a 5-HT disturbance – anxiety and aggression regulation are primarily disturbed, while mood lowering is a derivative symptom. Consequently, he expected that certain drugs such as L-tryptophan, the azapirones or lithium might ameliorate anxiety and/or aggression regulation via regulation of the 5-HT system to exert in addition an overall therapeutic effect in depression. Supposing van Praag's concept would hold true, one may speculate that lithium might also possess acute antisuicidal properties. A recently approved clinical project at the Department of Psychiatry, University of Dresden, will address this pressing question [68].

It is unfortunate that only few experimental psychologists tried to integrate the clinical effects of lithium into psychological constructs of experience and behavior as well as of cognition. Thus, some experimental approaches of the Berlin group, including the backward masking technique, and refined EEG studies point to a lithium-induced restricted number of degrees of freedom in neuropsychological/neurophysiological terms which might be related to a shorter persistence of external and internal stimuli. Such effects of long-term lithium medication might also fit to the observation derived from memory experiments in healthy volunteers that short-term administration of lithium modifies (diminishes) spontaneous initial action or, in other words, the will to act [69–73].

The second intriguing question associated with the issue of specificity is whether the antisuicidal effect of lithium would also occur in patients not responding optimally in terms of episode prevention. Part of the IGSLI data does in fact support such a concept. Addressing this issue, Ahrens and Müller-Oerlinghausen [74] selected only patients with at least 1 suicide attempt in the past before the onset of lithium medication (n = 176; 55% bipolar, 18% schizoaffective). The sample was divided into three subgroups according to their response to lithium long-term treatment in terms of reduction of depressive inpatient episodes. Despite the clearly different overall efficacy of lithium prophylaxis a statistically significant reduction of suicide attempts occurred in all three groups, even in the poor responders who did not show a significant decrease in the depressive inpatient episodes. In other words, in 50% of the clear-cut nonresponders no further suicide attempt was observed during lithium treatment. The standardized suicide mortality in the poor responders was 17.0 compared to an expected figure of approximately 100.

Certainly, these findings can neither prove the suicide-preventive effect of lithium nor its potential specificity. However, the accumulated evidence strongly supports such a possibility.

Studies on Potential Antisuicidal Effects of Lithium as a Trace Element in Drinking Water

Much scientific and media attention has been raised by recent epidemiological studies hinting at the possibility that even extremely low amounts of lithium could exert antisuicidal and antiaggressive effects. There exist at present 5 studies – 4 positive and 1 negative – linking lithium levels in drinking water to suicide rates in various countries and regions. Of these, 2 studies, 1 from Japan [75] and the other from Austria [76, 77], concluded that areas with higher lithium levels in the drinking water had lower suicide rates. A Greek study by Giotakos et al. [78] confirmed these results, as the authors found a tendency for lower suicide rates in the prefectures with high levels of lithium in drinking water. Blüml et al. [79] also showed in a state-wide sample of 3,123 lithium measurements in the public water supply of Texas that lithium levels were negatively associated with suicide rates in most statistical analyses.

A study by Kabacs et al. [80] measuring lithium levels in tap water in 47 subdivisions of the East of England and correlating these with the respective suicide SMR in each subdivision did not show an association between lithium level in drinking water and suicide rates.

Very recently, these studies were summarized and reviewed by Vita et al. [81]. The authors conclude that 'their results are surprisingly consistent in demonstrating a highly significant correlation between lithium levels in drinking water and suicide rates'.

To the knowledge of the authors, so far no pharmacological or biochemical findings exist which could be attributed to these fascinating and provocative findings, the interpretation of which, however, has to consider the usual pitfalls of any epidemiological data.

The Efficiency of Lithium Prophylaxis in Terms of Saved Lives
In 2004, Joffe [82] posed the question in an editorial: 'Does lithium save lives?' Ahrens and Müller-Oerlinghausen [83] developed a model for the calculation of deaths and suicides to be expected in the general population and in untreated patients with affective disorders. Based on their calculation they concluded that 5 suicides per year and 1,000 treated patients can be prevented. This would result in approximately 250 suicides per year prevented in Germany. The IGSLI data also shows that the average age of patients having committed suicide was 44. Thus, the gain for the gross national product in Germany would be 3,060 working years before completing the age of 65.

Clozapine

Clozapine Counteracts Suicidality and Aggressive Behavior in Patients with Schizophrenia and Borderline Personality Disorder
The risk of suicide exists not only in patients with mood disorders but also in those with a diagnosis of schizophrenia and schizoaffective and borderline personality disorders (BPD). It is said that suicide accounts for approximately 10% of deaths in patients with schizophrenia [84–86]. About one third will attempt suicide at least once in their life. Various clinical trials have shown that clozapine is unique among all antipsychotic agents as it can reduce positive as well as negative symptoms in schizophrenic patients not responding to any other typical or atypical neuroleptic medication. According to the recent guideline of the European Psychiatric Association on suicide prevention clozapine is also effective in reducing suicidal behavior in schizophrenic patients [87]. Corresponding evidence appears to be much weaker for any other 'atypical' antipsychotics such as olanzapine, risperidone or quetiapine.

Besides many case reports, there exist also some controlled prospective studies which have been summarized by Aguilar and Siris [86] and Kerwin and Bolonna [85]. A prospective but noncontrolled study by Meltzer and Okayli [88] as well as a retrospective study by Walker et al. [89] strongly suggested that clozapine can dramatically reduce the number of suicides and suicide attempts. A large independent multicenter, international RCT on 980 patients over 2 years (the International Suicide Prevention Trial Study in collaboration with the FDA) could then clearly demonstrate that clozapine was about 25% superior to olanzapine in preventing suicidal acts [90].

Already in 1998, Meltzer [84] recommended from the then existing evidence that clozapine should not only be prescribed to antipsychotic drug nonresponders but also to responders showing persistent suicidal thoughts and behavior – which would actually be an off-label use of this compound.

Clozapine did not show special superiority in antisuicidal activity among a group of atypical antipsychotics including olanzapine, risperidone or ziprasidone within a recently published nested case-control study from Sweden [91]. Interestingly, the authors could not identify any antisuicidal activity for antipsychotic depot injections nor for antidepressants or lithium administered to 4,000 schizophrenic and schizoaffective patients, including 84 patients who died by suicide within 5 years of diagnosis.

Treatment of Aggressive and Self-Mutilating Behavior in Patients with Borderline Personality Disorder

Suicidal, self-mutilating and aggressive behavior often poses serious problems in the care of patients with BPD. According to Paris and Zweig-Frank [92] approximately 10% of patients with BPD die from suicide. A multitude of case reports in the past have suggested that clozapine acts very favorably in such patients since it reduces self-injurious as well as open aggressive behavior. Zarzar and McEvoy [93] support the existing evidence by adding 4 very impressive cases of BPD patients having been admitted, often repeatedly, to a state hospital. All of them received clozapine (with blood levels ranging between 161 and 312 ng/ml). The striking and obvious results of the medication were as follows: (1) the reduction of self-injurious behavior appeared in a short time, i.e. within 2 weeks, (2) patients reported a 'marked reduction in misery' and (3) the need of restrictive measures (restraining, 1:1 observation) could be reduced mostly within a few weeks.

As mentioned above, a general more or less unique antipsychotic effectiveness of clozapine which also possesses antidepressant activity is observed when it comes to the treatment of schizophrenic patients unresponsive to medication with other antipsychotics. Thus, neurobiological findings suggesting specific pharmacological properties in which clozapine differs from other antipsychotics might perhaps provide some clues to the mechanism of the antisuicidal effect of lithium. In this context it appears to be of interest that on one side the activation of postsynaptic 5-HT_{1A} receptors in corticolimbic areas seems to be associated with the therapeutic effects of antidepressants, while on the other side characteristics of the postsynaptic receptors in the prefrontal cortex might be related to the unique properties of clozapine [94]. Clozapine is said to exert functional agonistic effects on these receptors in vivo, possibly resulting in increased dopamine release in the prefrontal cortex via activation of the mesocortical pathway. It has been speculated that this effect could be seen as a biological correlate to its beneficial effect on negative symptoms and cognitive deficits in chronic schizophrenic patients. Lithium, on the other hand, has also been shown to enhance 5-HT_{1A} receptor function, whereas chronic stress reduces the gene expression of these receptors in experimental animals. Increased 5-HT_{1A} receptor binding in the hippocampus and amygdala has also been shown in humans having been exposed to lithium medication [95].

References

1 Healy D, Whitaker C: Antidepressants and suicide: risk-benefit conundrums. J Psychiatry Neurosci 2003;28:331–337.
2 Holvey C, Connolly A, Taylor D: Psychiatric side effects of non-psychiatric drugs. Brit J Hospital Med 2010;1:432–436.
3 Stübner S, Grohmann R, v. Strahelndorff I, Rüther E, Möller HJ, Müller-Oerlinghausen B, Engel RR, Horvath A, Greil W: Suicidality as rare adverse event of antidepressant medication: report from the AMSP multicenter drug safety surveillance project. J Clin psychiatry 2010;71:1293–1307.
4 Müller-Oerlinghausen B: Suizidales Verhalten als unerwünschte Arzneimittelwirkung. Suizidprophylaxe 2014;41:106–112.
5 Oxenkrug G, Turski W, Zgraika W, Weinstock J, Ruthazer R, Summergrad P: Disturbances of tryptophan metabolism and risk of depression in HCV patients treated with IFN-α. J Infect Dis Ther 2014; 2:131.
6 Menke A, Domschke K, Czamara D, Klengel T, Hennings J, Lucae S, Baune BT, Arolt V, Müller-Myhsok B, Holsboer F, Binder EB: Genome-wide association study of antidepressant treatment-emergent suicidal ideation. Neuropsychopharmacology 2012;37:797–807.
7 Bschor T, Müller-Oerlinghausen B: Antidepressiva verringern nicht das Risiko von Suiziden oder Suizidversuchen bei depressiven Patienten. Arzneiverord Prax 2014;41:2–5.
8 Fergusson D, Doucette S, Glass KC, Shapiro S, Healy D, Hutton B: Association between suicide attempts and selective serotonin uptake inhibitors: systematic review of randomised controlled studies. BMJ 2005; 330:396.
9 Gibbons RD, Brown CD, Hur K, Davis J, Mann JJ: Suicidal thoughts and behaviour with antidepressant treatment: reanalysis of the randomized placebo-controlled studies of fluoxetine and venlafaxine. Arch Gen Psychiatry 2012;69:580–587.
10 Lewitzka U, Severus E, Bauer R, Ritter P, Müller-Oerlinghausen B, Bauer M: The suicide protective effects of lithium: more than 20 years of evidence. Int J Bipolar Dis, in press.
11 Tsuang MT, Woolson RF: Excess mortality in schizophrenia and affective disorders. Do suicides and accidental deaths solely account for this excess? Arch Gen Psychiatry 1978;35:1181–1185.
12 Weeke A: Causes of death in manic depressives; in Schou M, Strömgren E (eds): Origin, Prevention and Treatment of Affective Disorders. London, Academic Press, 1979, pp 289–299.
13 Hagnell O, Lanke J, Rorsman B: Suicide rates in the Lundby study: mental illness as a risk factor for suicide. Neuropsychobiology 1981;7:248–253.
14 Tuckman J, Youngman W: Identifying suicide with groups among attempted suicide. Public Health Rep 1963;78:763–766.
15 Motto I: Suicide attempts: a longitudinal view. Arch Gen Psychiatry 1965;13:516–520.
16 Guze SB, Robins E: Suicide in primary affective disorders. Br J Psychiatry 1970;117:437–438.
17 Goodwin FK, Jamison KR: Manic-depressive illness. New York, Oxford University Press, 1990.
18 WHO: Preventing Suicide: A Resource for General Physicians. Geneva, WHO, 2000. http://www.who.int/mental_health/media/en/56.pdf?ua=1.
19 Isometsä E: Suicidal behaviour in mood disorders – who, when, and why? Can J Psychiatry 2014;59:120–130.
20 Harris EC, Barraclough B: Excess mortality of mental disorder. Br J Psychiatry 1998;173:11–53.
21 Ahrens B, Müller-Oerlinghausen B, Schou M, Wolf T, Alda M, Grof E, Grof P, Lenz G, Simhandl C, Thau K, Wolf R, Möller HJ: Excess cardiovascular and suicide mortality of affective disorders may be reduced by lithium-prophylaxis. J Affect Disord 1995;33:67–75.
22 Barraclough B: Suicide prevention, recurrent affective disorder and lithium. Br J Psychiatry 1972;121: 391–392.
23 Müller-Oerlinghausen B, Müser-Causemann B, Volk J: Suicides and parasuicides in a high-risk patient group on and off lithium long-term medication. J Affect Disord 1992;25:261–270.
24 Felber W, Kyber A: Suizide und Parasuizide während und ausserhalb einer Lithiumprophylaxe; in Müller-Oerlinghausen B, Berghöfer A (eds): Ziele und Ergebnisse der medikamentösen Prophylaxe affektiver Psychosen. Stuttgart/New York, Thieme, 1994, pp 53–59.
25 Coppen A, Standish-Barry H, Bailey J, Houston G, Silcocks P, Hermon C: Does lithium reduce the mortality of recurrent mood disorders? J Affect Disord 1991;23:1–7.
26 Ahrens B, Müller-Oerlinghausen B: Einfluss der Lithiumprophylaxe auf die Mortalität von affektiven Psychosen; in Lungershausen E, Kaschka WP, Witkowsli RJ (eds): Affektive Psychosen. Stuttgart/New York, Schattauer, 1990, pp 334–337.
27 Coppen A: Depression as a lethal disease: prevention strategies. J Clin Psychiatry 1994;55:37–45.
28 Müller-Oerlinghausen B, Ahrens B, Grof E, Grof P, Lenz G, Schou M, Simhandl C, Thau K, Volk J, Wolf R, Wolf T: The effect of long-term lithium treatment on the mortality of patients with manic-depressive and schizo-affective illness. Acta Psychiatr Scand 1992;86:218–222.

29 Müller-Oerlinghausen B, Wolf T, Ahrens B, Schou M, Grof E, Grof P, Lenz G, Simhandl C, Thau K, Wolf R: Mortality during initial and during later lithium treatment: a collaborative study by IGSLI. Acta Psychiatr Scand 1994;90:295–297.

30 Bocchetta A, Ardau R, Burrai C, Chillotti C, Quesada G, del Zompo M: Suicidal behaviour on and off lithium prophylaxis in a group of patients with prior suicide attempts. J Clin Psychopharmacol 1998;18:384–389.

31 Baldessarini RJ, Tondo L, Hennen J: Effects of lithium treatment and its discontinuation on suicidal behavior in bipolar manic-depressive disorders. J Clin Psychiatry 1999;60:77–84.

32 Nilsson A: Mortality in recurrent mood disorders during periods on and off lithium. A complete population study in 362 patients. Pharmacopsychiatry 1995;28:8–13.

33 Schou M: The effect of prophylactic lithium treatment on mortality and suicidal behavior: a review for clinicians. J Affect Disord 1998;50:253–259.

34 Kallner G, Lindelius R, Petterson U, Stockman O, Tham A: Mortality in 497 patients with affective disorders attending a lithium clinic of after having left it. Pharmacopsychiatry 2000;33:8–13.

35 Angst J, Angst F, Gerber-Werder R, Gamma A: Suicide in mood-disorder patients with and without long-term medication: a 40 to 44 years' follow-up. Arch Suicide Res 2005;9:279–300.

36 Vestergaard P, Aagaard J: Five-year mortality in lithium-treated manic-depressive patients. J Affect Disord 1991;21:33–38.

37 Brodersen A, Licht RW, Vestergaard P, Olesen AV, Mortensen PB: Sixteen-year mortality in patients with affective disorder commenced on lithium. Br J Psychiatry 2000;176:429–433.

38 Coryell W, Arndt S, Turvey C, Endicott J, Solomon D, Mueller T, Leon AC, Keller M: Lithium and suicidal behaviour in major affective disorder: a case-control study. Acta Psychiatr Scand 2001;104:193–197.

39 Tondo L, Jamison KR, Baldessarini RJ: Effect of lithium maintenance on suicidal behavior in major mood disorders. Ann N Y Acad Sci 1997;836:339–351.

40 Cipriani A, Pretty H, Hawton K, Geddes JR: Lithium in the prevention of suicidal behaviour and all-cause mortality in patients with mood disorders: a systematic review of randomized trials. Am J Psychiatry 2005;162:1805–1819.

41 Cipriani A, Hawton K, Stockton S, Geddes JR: Lithium in the prevention of suicide in mood disorders: updated systematic review and meta-analysis. BMJ 2013;346:f3646.

42 Baldessarini RJ, Tondo L, Davis P, Pompili M, Goodwin FK, Hennen J: Decreased risk of suicides and attempts during long-term lithium treatment: a meta-analytic review. Bipolar Disord 2006;8:625–639.

43 Lauterbach E, Felber W, Müller-Oerlinghausen B, Ahrens B, Bronisch T, Meyer T, Kilb B, Lewitzka U, Hawellek B, Quante A, Richter K, Brooks A, Hohagen F: Adjunctive lithium treatment in the prevention of suicidal behaviour in depressive disorders: a randomised, placebo-controlled, 1-year trial. Acta Psychiatr Scand 2008;118:469–479.

44 Rombold F, Lauterbach E, Felber W, Müller-Oerlinghausen B, Ahrens B, Bronisch T, Kilb B, Lewitzka U, Richter K, Brooks A, Heuser I, Hohagen F, Quante A: Adjunctive lithium treatment in the prevention of suicidal behaviour in patients with depression and comorbid personality disorder. Int J Psychiatry Clin Pract 2014;18:300–303.

45 Thies-Flechtner K, Müller-Oerlinghausen B, Seibert W, Walther A, Greil W: Effect of prophylactic treatment on suicide risk in patients with major affective disorders. Data from a randomized prospective trial. Pharmacopsychiatry 1996;29;103–107.

46 Greil W, Ludwig-Mayerhofer W, Erazo N, Schöchlin C, Schmidt S, Engel RR, Czernik A, Giedke H, Müller-Oerlinghausen B, Osterheider M, Rudolf GAE, Sauer H, Tegeler J, Wetterling T: Lithium versus carbamazepine in the maintenance treatment of bipolar disorders – a randomised study. J Affect Disord 1997;43:151–161.

47 Goodwin FK: Anticonvulsant therapy and suicide in affective disorders. J Clin Psychiatry 1999;60:89–93.

48 Goodwin FK, Fireman B, Simon GE, Hunkeler EM, Lee J, Revicki D: Suicide risk in bipolar disorder during treatment with lithium and divalproex. JAMA 2003;290:1467–1473.

49 Collins JC, McFarland BH: Divalproex, lithium and suicide among Medicaid patients with bipolar disorder. J Affect Disord 2008;107:23–28.

50 Oquendo MA, Galfalvy HC, Currier D, Grunebaum MF, Sher L, Sullivan GM, Burke AK, Harkavy-Freedman J, Sublette ME, Parsey RV, Mann JJ: Treatment of suicide attempters with bipolar disorder: a randomised clinical trial comparing lithium and valproate in the prevention of suicidal behaviour. Am J Psychiatry 2011;168:1050–1056.

51 Weisler RH, Nolen WA, Neijber A, Hellqvist A, Paulsson B; Trial 144 Study Investigators: Continuation of quetiapine versus switching to placebo or lithium for maintenance treatment of bipolar I disorder (trial 144; a randomized controlled study). J Clin Psychiatry 2011;72:1452–1464.

52 Khan A, Khan SR, Hobus J, Faucett J, Mehra V, Giller EL, Rudolph RL: Differential pattern of response in mood symptoms and suicide risk measures in severely ill depressed patients assigned to citalopram with placebo or citalopram combined with lithium: role of lithium levels. J Psychiatr Res 2011;45:1489–1496.

53 Baldessarini RJ, Tondo L, Hennen J: Reduced suicide risk during long-term treatment with lithium. Ann NY Acad Sci 2001;932:24–43.

54 Müller-Oerlinghausen B: Lithium long-term treatment – does it act via serotonin? Pharmacopsychiatry 1985;18:214–217.
55 Müller-Oerlinghausen B: Die Wirkung von Lithium auf serotoninerge Funktionen; in Müller-Oerlinghausen B, Greil W, Berghöfer A (eds): Die Lithiumtherapie. Berlin/Heidelberg/New York, Springer, 1997, pp 61–68.
56 Nilsson A: The anti-aggressive actions of lithium. Rev Contemp Pharmacother 1993;4:269–285.
57 Müller-Oerlinghausen B, Lewitzka U: Lithium reduces pathological aggression and suicidality: a mini-review. Neuropsychobiology 2010;62:43–49.
58 Ohmura Y, Tsutsui-Kimura I, Kumamoto H, Minami M, Izumi T, Yamaguchi T, Yoshida T, Yoshioka M: Lithium, but not valproic acid or carbamazepine, suppresses impulsive-like action in rats. Psychopharmacology 2012;219:421–432.
59 Kovacsics CE, Gould TD: Shock-induced aggression in mice is modified by lithium. Pharmacol Biochem Behav 2010;94:380–386.
60 Mühlbauer HD, Müller-Oerlinghausen B: Fenfluramine stimulation of serum cortisol in patients with major affective disorders and healthy controls: further evidence for a central serotonergic action of lithium in man. J Neural Transm 1985;61:81–94.
61 Steiner J, Bielau H, Brisch R, Danos P,Ullrich O, Mawrin C, Bernstein HG, Bogerts B: Immunological aspects in the neurobiology of suicide: elevated microglial density in schizophrenia and depression is associated with suicide. Psychiatr Res 2008;42:151–157.
62 Erhardt S, Lim CK, Linderholm KR, Janelidze S, Lindquist D, Samuelsson M, Lundberg K, Postolache TT, Träksman-Bendz L, Guillemin GJ, Brundin L: Connecting inflammation with glutamate agonism. Neuropsychopharmacology 2013;38:743–752.
63 Steiner J, Bogerts B, Samyai Z, Walter M, Gos T, Bernstein HG, Myint AM: Bridging the gap between the immune and glutamate hypotheses of schizophrenia and major depression: potential role of glial NMDA receptor modulators and impaired blood-brain barrier integrity. World J Biol Psychiatry 2012;13:437–492.
64 Kovacsics CE, Gottesman II, Gould TD: Lithium's antisuicidal efficacy: elucidation of neurobiological targets using endophenotype strategies. Ann Rev Pharmacol Toxicol 2009;49:175–198.
65 Linden M, Zäske H, Ahrens B: Correlates of suicidal ideation in general healthcare patients – results of the WHO Collaborative Study on Psychological Problems in General Health Care (WHO-PPGHC). Int J Psychiatry Clin Pract 2003;7:17–25.
66 Painuly N, Sharan P, Mattoo SK: Relationship of anger and anger attacks with depression: a brief review. Eur Arch Psychiatry Clin Neurosci 2005;255:215–222.
67 van Praag HM: Anxiety and increased aggression as pacemakers of depression. Acta Psychiatr Scand 1998;393:81–88.
68 Lewitzka U, Jabs B, Fülle M, Holthoff V, Juckel G, Uhl I, Kittel-Schneider S, Reif A, Reif-Leonhard C, Gruber O, Djawid B, Goodday S, Haussmann R, Pfennig A, Ritter P, Conell J, Severus E, Bauer M: Does lithium reduce suicidal ideation and behavior? A protocol for a randomized, placebo-controlled multicenter trial of lithium plus treatment as usual (TAU) in patients with suicidal major depressive episode. BMC Psychiatry 2015;15:117.
69 Kropf D, Müller-Oerlinghausen B: Changes in learning, memory, and mood during lithium treatment. Acta Psychiatr Scand 1979;59:97–124.
70 Kropf D, Müller-Oerlinghausen B: Effects of lithium on visual perception in manic depressive patients without acute symptomatology. Neuropsychobiology 1986;15:34–42.
71 Müller-Oerlinghausen B: Towards a neurophysiological model of the mode of action of lithium. Pharmacopsychiatry 1987;20:192–194.
72 Ulrich G, Herrmann WM, Hegerl U, Müller-Oerlinghausen B: Effects of lithium on the dynamics of electroencephalographic vigilance in healthy subjects. J Affect Disord 1990;20:19–25.
73 Classen W: Der psychologische Zugang zur Wirkungsweise von Lithium; in Müller-Oerlinghausen B, Greil W, Berghöfer A (eds): Die Lithiumtherapie. Nutzen, Risiken, Alternativen, ed 2. Berlin/Heidelberg/New York, Springer, 1997, pp 118–136.
74 Ahrens B, Müller-Oerlinghausen B: Does lithium exert an independent anti-suicidal effect? Pharmacopsychiatry 2001;34:132–136.
75 Ohgami H, Tero T, Shiotsuki I, Ishii N, Iwata N: Lithium levels in drinking water and risk of suicide. Br J Psychiatry 2009;194:464–465.
76 Kapusta ND, Mossaheb N, Etzersdorfer E, Hlavin G, Thau K, Willeit M, Praschak-Rieder N, Sonneck G, Leithner-Dziubas K: Lithium in drinking water and suicide mortality. Br J Psychiatry 2011;198:346–350.
77 Helbich M, Leithner M, Kapusta ND: Geospatial examination of lithium in drinking water and suicide mortality. Int J Health Geogr 2012;13:11–19.
78 Giotakos O, Nisianakis P, Tsouvelas G, Giakalou VV: Lithium in the public water supply and suicide mortality in Greece. Biol Trace Elem Res 2013;156:376–379.
79 Blüml V, Regier MD, Hlavin G, Rocket IR, König F, Vyssoki B, Bschor T, Kapusta ND: Lithium in the public water supply and mortality in Texas. J Psychiatr Res 2013;47:407–411.
80 Kabacs N, Memon A, Obinwa T, Stochl J, Perez J: Lithium in drinking water and suicide rates across the East of England. Br J Psychiatry 2011;198:406–407.

81 Vita A, de Peri L, Sacchetti E: Lithium in drinking water and suicide prevention: a review of the evidence. Int Clin Psychopharmacol 2015;30:1–5.
82 Joffe RT: Editorial: does lithium save lives? J Psychiatry Neurosci 2004;29:9.
83 Ahrens B, Müller-Oerlinghausen B: Die antisuizidale und mortalitätssenkende Wirkung von Lithium; in Müller-Oerlinghausen B, Greil W, Berghöfer A (eds): Die Lithiumtherapie. Berlin/Heidelberg/New York, Springer, 1997, pp 262–277.
84 Meltzer HY: Suicide in schizophrenia: risk factors and clozapine treatment. J Clin Psychiatry 1998;59: 15–20.
85 Kerwin RW, Bolonna AA: Is clozapine antisuicidal? Expert Rev Neurother 2004;4:187–190.
86 Aguilar EJ, Siris SG: Do antipsychotic drugs influence suicidal behavior in schizophrenia? Psychopharmacol Bull 2007;40:128–142.
87 Wasserman D, Rihmer Z, Rujescu D, Sarchiapone M, Sokolowski M, Titelman D, Zalsman G, Zemishlany Z, Carli V; European Psychiatric Association: The European Psychiatric Association (EPA) guidance on suicide treatment and prevention. Eur Psychiatry 2012;27:129–141.
88 Meltzer HY, Okayli G: Reduction of suicidality during clozapine treatment of neuroleptic-resistant schizophrenia: impact on risk-benefit assessment. Am J Psychiatry 1995;152:183–190.
89 Walker AM, Lanza LL, Arellano R, Rothman KJ: Mortality in current and former users of clozapine. Epidemiology 1997;8:671–677.
90 Meltzer HY, Alphs L, Green AI, Atamura AC, Anand R, Bertold A, Bourgeois M, Chouinard G, Islam MZ,Kane J, Krishnan R, Lendenmayer JP, Potkin S; International Suicide Prevention Trial Study Group: Clozapine treatment for suicidality in schizophrenia: International Suicide Prevention Trial (InterSePT). Arch Gen Psychiatry 2003;60:82–91.
91 Reutfors J, Bahmanyar S, Jönsson EG, Brandt L, Boden R, Ekbom A, Ösby U: Medication and suicide risk in schizophrenia: a nested case-control study. Schizophr Res 2013;150:416–420.
92 Paris J, Zweig-Frank H: A 27-year follow-up of patients with borderline personality disorder. Compr Psychiatry 2001;42:482–487.
93 Zarzar T, McEvoy J: Clozapine for self-injurious behavior in individuals with borderline personality disorder. Ther Adv Psychopharmacol 2013;3:272–274.
94 Celada P, Bortolozzi A, Artigas F: Serotonin 5-HT_{1A} receptors as targets for agents to treat psychiatric disorders: rationale and current status of research. CNS Drugs 2013;27:703–716.
95 Nugent AC, Carlson PJ, Bain EE, Eckelman W, Herscovitch P, Manji H, Zarate CA, Drevets WC: Mood stabilizer treatment increases serotonin type 1A receptor binding in bipolar depression. J Psychopharmacol 2013;27:894–902.

Prof. Dr. med. Bruno Müller-Oerlinghausen
Charité Universitäts-Medizin Berlin and Freie Universität Berlin
Bartningallee 11–13
DE–14050 Berlin (Germany)
E-Mail Bruno.mueller-oerlinghausen@web.de

Kaschka WP, Rujescu D (eds): Biological Aspects of Suicidal Behavior.
Adv Biol Psychiatry. Basel, Karger, 2016, vol 30, pp 161–163 (DOI: 10.1159/000439105)

Challenges for Future Research and Closing Remarks

Dan Rujescu[a] · Iris N. Kaschka[b] · Wolfgang P. Kaschka[c]

[a]Department of Psychiatry, Psychotherapy and Psychosomatics, University of Halle, Halle, [b]Department of Neuroradiology, University Hospital Erlangen, Erlangen, and [c]Department of Psychiatry and Psychotherapy I, University of Ulm, Zentrum für Psychiatrie Südwürttemberg, Ulm/Ravensburg, Germany

Current epidemiological data reveal that suicide is a prominent cause of death worldwide and represents a major health problem in modern societies. Beside psychopathological, psychosocial, economic, and cultural conditions, neurobiological factors have been shown to be involved in the causation of suicidal behaviour. A great number of in vivo and post mortem studies have been conducted to identify abnormalities in stress response via the hypothalamo-pituitary-adrenal axis and in a broad spectrum of neurotransmitter systems, above all the serotonergic, noradrenergic and GABAergic systems. The fine tuning of these systems and their interplay in mood regulation and coping with environmental stress is not yet completely understood. The same is true of the regulatory processes controlling neuroplasticity and neurogenesis which appear to play an eminent role in psychiatric diseases like major depression or bipolar disorder and – most probably – also in suicidal behaviour.

It has long been known that infectious and inflammatory processes of the central nervous system are often associated with a host of psychiatric conditions. Consequently, numerous investigators have focused their interest on immunological processes in psychiatric diseases. Working with behavioural intermediate phenotypes such as impulsivity, aggression or hopelessness, rather than suicidal behaviour, appears to open up new avenues of research enabling us to dissect a complex behaviour into well-defined components which may be more easily accessible to empirical studies. To learn more about the crosstalk of the different components of the immune system via cytokines, neurotrophic factors and others, as well as its contribution to neuroplasticity and its intricate links with neurotransmitter systems, will be a big task for future research and a promising field for the development of novel therapeutic interventions, including suicide preventive measures.

The last few years have brought about an explosion of interest in genomics. Genome-wide association studies analyse more than one million genetic variants at once. Furthermore, exome and whole genome sequencing projects have already started. All these new studies will help us to further characterize genetic risk factors of suicidal behaviour. Interestingly, many of these risk factors are also associated with personality traits like impulsivity or aggression. These genetic variants have raised a number of fascinating new clinical and scientific questions, especially concerning the phenotypic boundaries between mental disorders as they are currently classified and their modes of inheritance, as well as the implications of this new information for diagnostics and genetic counselling.

The relative contributions of heritable versus environmental risk factors to suicidal behaviour will remain a challenging research issue in the future – all the more since we have just begun to gain some insight into the fascinating role of epigenetics in the gene-environment interaction.

During the last decades, we have witnessed huge progress in structural and functional neuroimaging technologies. Just to name the most important techniques: computerized tomography, single photon emission computed tomography, positron emission computed tomography (PET) with an ever-increasing number of radioligands, magnetic resonance imaging (MRI) including functional MRI, MRI spectroscopy, diffusion tensor imaging, and finally, recent hybrid techniques (MRI and PET combined in one device). These techniques in all their modifications enable us to observe the brain in vivo, not only with regard to structure but also during functional tasks or the processing of well-defined stimuli. To measure regional blood flow or glucose utilization, to visualize the binding of ligands to specific receptors and to trace psychopharmacological compounds at their site of action – by choosing the appropriate technology all of these tasks are likewise feasible. Applied to suicide research, it may be expected that these tools will enable us to further our understanding of the pathophysiology of suicidal behaviour and extend our repertoire of preventive measures.

A small number of psychopharmacological compounds proved to possess suicide-prophylactic efficacy. This feature was first described in lithium salts, and they are still the most widely used and prominent representatives of this group. Lithium is known to exert its effects – at least in part – via the inositol phosphate second messenger system and to influence neuroplasticity. On the other hand, a better understanding of the pathophysiological mechanisms involved in suicidal behaviour could enable us to reveal the mechanism of action of compounds like lithium salts, the antisuicidal efficacy of which has been demonstrated in numerous studies. Some recent studies indicate that lithium treatment might be associated with better decision-making performance in bipolar patients. If these findings can be replicated, similar studies would be warranted in patients with a history of suicide attempts or being at risk of suicide. Furthermore, the issue of an antisuicidal effect of lithium salts occurring as trace elements in drinking water is not yet finally settled, so that further studies appear to be warranted also in this field.

To develop sufficiently sensitive and specific tools for the assessment of suicide risk in individual persons, an integrated approach will be necessary comprising not only clinical examination, thorough psychiatric exploration, and neuropsychological testing but also biological test procedures contributed by the disciplines of genetics/epigenetics, molecular biology, biochemistry, electrophysiology, psychoneuroimmunology, neuroimaging, and possibly others. As a perspective for the future, one might speculate that the integration of results obtained in the above-mentioned areas of research could be utilized to construct an algorithm or 'suicide risk index' which might be helpful in improving suicide risk assessment and suicide prevention.

Prof. Dr. Wolfgang P. Kaschka
Department of Psychiatry and Psychotherapy I
University of Ulm, Zentrum für Psychiatrie Südwürttemberg
Weingartshofer Strasse 2, DE–88214 Ravensburg (Germany)
E-Mail wolfgang.kaschka@zfp-zentrum.de

Author Index

Subject Index